Self Cure

YOU CAN DO MORE
FOR YOUR HEALTH
THAN YOUR DOCTOR CAN

Mark J. Sicherman, M.D.
with Chuck Stormon

Also by Mark J. Sicherman, M.D.
Levels of Consciousness
(medical short stories)

DEDICATION

For Dani and Gyata

CONTENTS

INTRODUCTION

How do you know if this book will be helpful to you? Ask yourself the following questions and if you answer yes to all or most of them, you will find what you are looking for in these pages.

Are you fed up with the one-size-fits-all impersonal approach of the medical profession?

Are you suffering from a chronic or recurrent condition that has not been responsive to prescription medications or surgery?

Are you looking for a more natural approach to healing, even if it requires time and effort on your part?

Do you find truth in the time-honored adage that an ounce of prevention is worth a pound of cure?

Do you value physical and emotional well-being more than the acquisition of wealth and power?

In the developed nations, most of us are born healthy. And we can remain healthy throughout our lives if we make the right choices. That is what the first part of this book is about - choosing a life-style that allows time for health-promoting and disease-preventing behaviors. Real preventive medicine is not about immunizations, yearly physicals and so-called early detection through endless lab tests and procedures. It is about taking charge of your own health and well-being, putting your SELF in your own hands, caring for yourself.

It is estimated that 75-80% of the visits made to doctors' offices are for diseases or conditions that are either self-limited (will heal in time without intervention) or that result from poor life-style choices. It is unrealistic to expect any health care system to rescue us from our excesses or our sick-making behaviors.

Physicians are for the most part well-meaning individuals. They will try to help us. They are trained to use the tools of their trade, the knife or the prescription blank, which are the wrong tools for getting the job done for most of what ails us. Application of those tools, while sometimes providing short-term relief of symptoms (after all, someone is doing something for us and that always makes us feel better), often leads to a worsening of our overall health down the road.

There are times in our lives when many of us will have a real need for medical intervention. Accidents happen. Severe infection can attack even the healthiest among us. Sometimes emergency surgery is required. The medical profession is adept at handling these life-threatening situations and seems to become more proficient at it with each passing decade.

For the past fifty years I have been a practicing member of what I used to consider a noble and immensely rewarding profession. But in the past few decades I have witnessed the overall quality of medicine in this country decline to the point where the whole system is now in crisis. While I have strong opinions about the policies and politics that led to this deplorable situation, this book is not the place to air them. This is not a book about healing the medical profession. Rather, what I hope is that my experience with patients and with my own health issues will be helpful to you in your quest to get healthy and stay that way.

The recommendations in this book are not based primarily on scientific studies. Medical research has been a disappointment to me, especially in recent years. Contradictory evidence abounds. Many drugs and procedures that proved effective in the 1970's and 80's are now found to be useless or harmful. Current drugs and procedures are promoted as scientific fact, but they may also be found ineffective or harmful in time.

Most doctors have become experts in specific disease entities of specific organ systems. Every patient who has a particular disease will be treated the same way. In contrast, my expertise has been in helping people to get to know themselves on a body/mind level. When a person achieves this self-awareness, they will know what they need in order to restore and maintain health. The self-care methods advanced in this book are valuable tools to use in this process. This is the science of Self-Cure.

This book is organized into the following three parts:

Part I: The Three Pillars of Good Health: Intake, Exercise, and Going to the Source;

Part II: Self Cure of Specific Problems; and

Part III: Resources for Self Cure.

It is important to read the first section before looking for relief of your symptoms in the second section. The body is not an automobile. There are no quick fixes. If you are basically unhealthy, trying to get specific symptom relief, while not harmful, will at best provide transient help. If you are following a health-enhancing life-style and develop some problem or condition in spite of all your efforts, Part II of the book will enlarge your therapeutic 'tool kit.'

Please be patient with yourself. It will take you a few months to implement enough of the disease-preventing, health promoting behaviors outlined in this book to assure you life-long health and well-being. In very practical terms, I would estimate that it will take about one hour per day to transition to and maintain a healthy life-style. Is it worth an hour of your time each day? Only you can answer that question. I can promise you that if you do commit the time and energy, after several months it will no longer feel as if you are pressed for time or saddled with another onerous chore. It will simply be the way you have chosen to live your life.

1 MY JOURNEY FROM PATIENT TO DOCTOR

When I was a kid, my family and everyone else who was important in my world had the same doctor. His name was Harold Levine, MD, but we called him Dr. Buddy. He treated my father's ulcers, my mother's nerves, and my sister's injuries. But I was the one on whom he worked magic.

I was a 'sickly' child, a condition likely brought on by my mother's morbid fear that something terrible would happen to me[1]. Lying in bed with yet another bout of low-grade fever, chills and a stomach ache, I would hear my mother on the phone with Dr. Buddy. Then I would wait, hardly daring to breathe, until I heard the front door open, my mother's fearful, hushed words to

---

[1] My mother fears were understandable. She grew up motherless, her own mother having died giving birth to her. Her father, whom she worshipped, died when I was an infant, leaving my mother bereft. In addition, she was traumatized by the violent death of her beloved nephew at age three.

him, and then his heavy footfalls on the stairs up to my room.

I remember the rumpled blue suit, the rimless glasses, the big black bag, the contagious broad smile. Hey, Buddy, he'd say, advancing toward the bed, preceded by a reassuring scent of disinfectant soap. In the doorway, my mother prattled on about my symptoms and her fears, but he ignored her. He listened to me, he saw me, he touched me and by the time he announced to my mother that it was 'nothing serious, probably the grippe,' I was healed. Oh, he always left a little vial of pills and a few instructions but I was fine. I stayed in bed a few hours longer to please my mother, then resumed the life of a normal child.

As I grew up, I knew I wanted to be like Dr. Buddy. I wanted to know everything he knew, I wanted to help kids like me and yes, I wanted to be important. And of course my parents were thrilled that I wanted to be a doctor.

I chose pediatrics as my specialty because I felt comfortable and happy around children. I practiced pediatrics in the Army, in private practice and clinic settings for about 12 years. There was a self-disparaging joke among baby doctors back then that "grandmothers can handle most of what we see in the office." Gradually I came to recognize the truth of that aphorism. It was the 80% rule that was operating; most of the problems these children had were either self-limiting or stress and lifestyle related.

Even with regard to more serious conditions, I began to realize that often it was my comforting presence that brought relief. One night, on a house call to a child who was in respiratory distress with asthma, I prepared a 'shot' of epinephrine to administer. The little girl's mother was understandably frantic, so I took the child in my arms into another room, but before I could give the shot, the wheezing subsided to the point where the medicine was unnecessary. It was my first lesson in mind/body medicine.

I went on to study MindBody Medicine, at first informally through reading, workshops, lectures and seminars; and then in a more formal way by enrolling in the training program of the New York Society for Bioenergetic Analysis[2]. After five years of training, supervision and therapy, I was certified as a bioenergetic therapist. This was a life-altering experience, for me personally and for my practice. For the next 35 years I worked with adult patients, practicing with them the kind of medicine I am now writing about in this book.

When I was a young pediatrician, my work was not only informed by the seven years of training I'd had, but also in large measure by being blessed with four young children of my own. I was very involved with the "mothering" of the children and I learned a lot from our kids that was directly helpful in the office.

A few years later, after a sad and difficult divorce, I married a woman with five children. Two years after that, my kids came to live with me and that made nine under the same roof. I was not used to chaos; I

---

[2] This discipline, founded by the noted psychiatrist Alexander Lowen, MD, is based on the premise that as an individual's character (or personality) is formed, his responses to the traumas of everyday life become structured in the body, forming blocks to the free flow of energy and feeling, and ultimately leading to disease states. Thus the therapeutic approach involves working with the body as well as the mind, in order to safely open these constricted areas and facilitate freedom of movement and expression.

struggled to maintain order in the house and in my psyche. I was in survival mode, dragging myself from home to work and trying to manage my developing psychosomatic illnesses. If not for that anguished era of my life, I would never have discovered the health restoring, sanity saving benefits of meditation. It has been 38 years since I learned to meditate and I have practiced it every day since then.

In my quest to restore my own health and to enhance my interventions with my patients, I encountered many gifted healers: psychotherapists, body workers, acupuncturists and physicians. When I learned techniques that worked well for me, such as meditation or breath exercises or eating healthy foods, I was eager to try them with my patients. In turn, the feedback that I got from patients in regard to a particular suggestion was most useful in determining which approaches I should add to my 'tool kit' (known in medical parlance as the therapeutic armamentarium). And now they have formed the basis of Parts II and III of this book.

My wife and I still live on our beautiful farm which she found for us nearly forty years ago. Our children and our pets and the land and the seasons have been remarkable teachers. Whatever wisdom I have gained I owe as much to them as to my more formal, structured training and experience. Our sixteen grandchildren provide ample opportunity for me to keep in practice as physician and therapist and as an observer of the human condition. In turn, they teach me about love and acceptance.

If there is a broader vision to this book, it goes something like this. I grew up thinking of medicine as a noble profession, and that is the way I practiced, without giving a lot of thought to the business end of it. I wouldn't have it any other way. Now there are signs (literally) reminding us that medicine is big business and highly competitive. More and more the main determinant of standard of care is the bottom line in a business sense. This problem is systemic; it is not the fault of the individual health care practitioner.

This state of affairs is sad, not just for the patients, but for the doctors as well, most of whom are missing out on the joy of helping the individual sitting before them, the whole human being who has put him or herself in their hands. I dare to hope that my efforts in creating this book will help to restore medicine to its proper place as a profession.

PART I

THE THREE PILLARS OF GOOD HEALTH

2 GETTING TO KNOW YOU

Omniscient in your juggler's booth
All is discovered through your patter
Except the simple obvious truth
Of what was actually the matter.
- Anonymous

Health is an individual matter. No one can give you specific advice about your health unless they are intimately acquainted with you – with your body and mind and spirit. You are unlikely to find any health professional, conventional or alternative, who can understand you that well. Healers with those skills do exist, but most of us do not have the time or resources to locate them. And I have found that the so-called healers who make a public display of their abilities are usually charlatans and should be avoided.

But there is someone who can get to know you well-enough to make intelligent decisions about your path to good health and well-being. That person is YOU. Although it requires a commitment of time, in the long run you will save a bundle of money. If you are not paying your own way, you will be saving taxpayer dollars, an act of kindness toward future generations.

So if I'm right about health being an individual matter, how do I have the audacity to write this book that tells you how to get healthy and stay that way? After all, I don't know you. I know nothing about how you think, what your beliefs are or what feelings possess you, let alone your current state of health. There are hundreds, perhaps thousands, of books written each year by people who want to tell you how to lose weight, become fit, avoid cancer, cure cancer and become a better person. Many of them are written by experts in their field, and some of them are helpful to some of the readers who 'stick with the program.'

Almost everyone I know, including myself, has at some time in their life found a book (or CD, DVD, website) which has been helpful to them in their quest for good health. When we find a self-help book we are excited about, we recommend it to our friends, relatives and co-workers. And we are disappointed at how few of them get on board. Most won't even read it. They're on a different path, even if we are sure that path will lead them to self-destruct.

As I cautioned in the opening words of the Introduction, this book is not for everyone. It is for those who are committed to getting healthy and staying that way. But still the question is, how can I help you do that if I do not know you? And the answer is that by helping you get to know yourself, to become intimate with your own mind, body and spirit, you will find the path that is right *for you*.

We all know men and women who lead grossly unhealthy life-styles and live to be centenarians. It is tempting to observe these people and say, "Why should

I have to exercise, give up certain foods and habits and curtail life's pleasures when my Uncle Al lived to be 100 smoking, drinking and eating junk every day?" How can they get away with that? I'm not sure. Good genes? Perhaps. In any case, you are probably more like me and don't have superhuman genes. If so, then Uncle Al's lifestyle will be detrimental to your health and longevity. So read on.

There are three pillars that provide the foundation for a healthy life. The first is Intake, which is nutrition plus everything else you take in. The second is Exercise. The third is Going to the Source.

Underlying these pillars are our relationships: community, family, friends and loved ones. These are essential for most of us as we follow the path of improving health and preventing disease. Interpersonal relationships are a necessary part of life for almost everyone on the planet. Research shows that the quality of our relationships with significant others can have powerful positive or negative effects on our health. I believe we should constantly strive to improve our relationships with family, friends, co-workers and the community at large. Feeling connected to others is salutary to our health and well-being.

This book is about Self-Cure, so I have not included a section on interpersonal relationships. There are numerous books on healing difficult relationships and individual or group therapy can be very helpful. I think you will find that by improving your state of health and well-being through the techniques advanced in this book, your relationships with others will also become stronger and more satisfying. You will find the section on Going to the Source to be most helpful in this regard.

3 THE FIRST PILLAR - INTAKE

*Our doctors eat the melon and drink the new
wine while they keep their patient tied down to
syrups and slops.*
- Michel de Montaigne

You can substitute the word Nutrition for Intake as
long as you agree with me that everything we *take in*,
through our lungs and skin and ears and eyes, as well as
our mouths, constitutes our nutritional input. You've
heard people say 'feast your eyes on this,' when they
present you with a visual treat. Most people would
rather look at a sunset than a pile of garbage. And most
of us would rather smell a rose than a pile of garbage.
But alas, there are too many of us who would choose to
eat a pile of garbage rather than consume a nutritious
meal.

If someone had tried to convince me 30 years ago
that soon we would all go around drinking water from a
bottle, I wouldn't have believed it. Yes, our water is
polluted. The air we breathe is polluted. The food we

eat is polluted. And most of the stuff we choose to listen to and look at on a daily basis amounts to visual and auditory pollution.

It is not good nutrition to sit down to a meal of organic rice and veggies while we are talking or texting on our cell phones or plopped in front of the TV watching people fight with each other or, for that matter if we are fighting with our spouses or yelling at our kids. Organic food is preferable to a meal of fast food or any other pile of garbage, but it's not going to ensure good health and well being.

Try this experiment, just once, no matter how busy you are. Buy an organic apple. Wash it well (organic does not mean germ-free) and carry it to a quiet spot next to a babbling brook. Sit and eat the apple slowly, chewing each bite fully. Notice when you choose to swallow. Complete each mouthful before taking another bite. Listen to the brook and look at the trees as you consume the apple. When finished, sit for a moment longer and ask yourself this question: "Do I feel well-nourished, at least right now?"

If you pay close attention to what you take in, on all the levels we have mentioned, you will slowly learn what needs to be done. I do not expect you to immediately stop eating in front of the TV or cease yelling at unruly kids or install air purifiers in every room in the house or go sit by a babbling brook in order to find peace of mind (and heart and belly). You will learn, as you read on, how to pay close attention to what you are doing in all aspects of your life, little bits at a time. And once you have given your life your full attention, your eyes and ears and your mind and mouth will serve as your guides on this path to good health.

Air. Water. Food. Noise. It's easy to feel overwhelmed, to give up and chow down a Big Mac. OK, fine. Just do it with awareness and with a realization that you can balance this later with healthy food. Rest assured that one meal loaded with trans fats and high fructose corn syrup will not give you cancer. One bottle of spring water in cheap plastic as you dash for the five-forty will not destroy your liver. But consuming garbage on a daily basis, combined with breathing the exhaust from fossil fuels, combined with overwork and no exercise, well, now you're courting disaster.

But there is no need to feel overwhelmed. Use the following information in this chapter as a guide. Here you will find small steps that you can take to improve your 'nutrition' without adding stress to your life. Choose the suggestions that attract you and seem easy. Soon you will find your health and your life improving, giving you incentive to make further changes.

Water

We now know that we need to be concerned not only about the purity of our water, but also the safety of the container. Rather than worrying about which type of plastic is safe and will not leach harmful chemicals into your water, switch to glass bottles. Buy a few 16 ounce bottles (bottled teas or juices from a natural foods store are a good source of these containers), fill them with water from a safe source and keep them in your car, backpack, on your desk at work.

Now you are wondering 'what is a safe source of water.' I trust the following: the five gallon glass jugs that can be delivered to your home by a reputable supplier; a refill station at your local natural food store;

or, water from the kitchen spigot of a friend who is lucky enough to have annually tested well water (free water is nice). If you can afford it, you can also have installed in your home a complete filtration system – just be sure that you keep it well-maintained.

You do not need to drink as much water as you have been led to believe by most health gurus. With the exception of the elderly, it is quite difficult to become dehydrated under normal circumstances. Unless you are exercising vigorously, you can wait until you get home to drink water. Drink when you are thirsty. But also consider that your mouth might feel dry for reasons other than thirst: dry air, prescription and over-the-counter medications, mouth breathing and fear.

We have been conditioned to believe that we must drink something at each meal. You do not need liquids while eating a meal. A glass of wine before dinner may aid digestion. But drinking water, soda, or other liquids throughout your meal dilutes digestive enzymes needed to process the food. When the server asks, "What would you like to drink with your meal?" it is preferable to say, "Nothing, thank you."

Air

Ideally, move to a rural location at high elevation and spend a lot of time outside in the fresh air. Alas, it is almost impossible for most of us to have any control over the quality of outside air that we breathe. We can elect officials who profess to have a genuine concern with environmental pollution and hope for the best, for our kids if not for ourselves.

But we can and should concern ourselves with the quality of our *indoor* air, because that is where we spend most of our time. I worry most about people who work in sealed environments and live in newer houses with air-tight insulation. If you have a choice, open a window at work and home. If not, and if you work in what you consider is a 'sick' building, go outside often. Also, buy a small air purifier or ionizer and keep it running on your desk. At home, especially if you live in a newer house, it is worth the additional heating expense to open several windows a bit to maintain cross-ventilation. There are also several varieties of effective air purifiers on the market. And while you are at it, maintain your indoor humidity at between 30-50%. You will notice the difference – less cough and congestion and fewer upper respiratory infections (see specifics in Part II).

Please remember that you do not need to feel overwhelmed by the suggestions for finding clean water to drink and air to breathe. Take your time. There is no rush. Disease states related to the intake of impure air and water take a long time to develop. Even if it takes you a year to implement the suggested changes, that's fine. The psychological stress of taking on too much at once is more harmful to your body than less-than-ideal air and water. Naturally, if you already have symptoms related to pollution (for example, asthma from smog or infection from contaminated water) you will need to act more quickly.

Medication

I consider the consumption of most prescription and over-the-counter medications hazardous to your health. In order to understand this, let us look more deeply into the '80% rule' that I mentioned in the Introduction. It is well-known that approximately eighty percent of the problems and conditions for which people seek medical help are either self-limited or are diseases of life-style. If the condition is self-limited, that is, it will resolve by itself in time, you do not need medication. If the problem is related to life-style, then you need behavioral changes to reverse the disease process and give your body the opportunity and time to heal itself.

I am not suggesting that you learn to suffer in silence. My friends and family know that I am not a stoic. Like me, while you are waiting impatiently for your self-limited illness to resolve itself or are getting fed-up with the very slow process of life-style change, you will desire and deserve symptom relief. But for the most part, we do not need to take medications to obtain relief. In Part II you will learn how to use food, exercise and the power of the mind/body connection to alleviate symptoms.

Eating well over a long period of time can greatly improve your health and solve a host of problems. If you are already taking medications regularly, you may be able to reduce the dosage or completely eliminate your intake of certain medications by altering your diet. Do not change your dosage without consulting your doctor first. Certain foods interact with medication, so be careful of how any drugs you are taking may be affected by changes in your diet.

It may be necessary at times for you to take prescription medications, especially if your condition falls into the 20% category which requires expert medical intervention. But it is very important that the prescribing process be individualized – one size does not fit all. People react very differently to medications, and this is especially true as we get older. Most doctors and other health care providers do not have time to pay attention to this phenomenon. Usually, if you have the same condition as the patient who just left the office, you will be given the same medication by the doctor, perhaps with some adjustment of the dosage based on your weight.

Of course you can not know if you will react badly to a drug until you try it, which is why it is very important – I would say essential – to take only one new medication at a time. Others, if necessary, can be added after a few days or weeks if you are able to tolerate the initial drug. It is well-known that the more medications you take in combination, the more likely you are to become seriously ill from potential drug interactions. It is reported that upwards of 100,000 people die annually from prescription drug interactions.

If you are taking a prescribed medication and you experience side-effects, your doctor will often prescribe another drug to counteract the side-effects of the initial medication. I consider this practice, despite its wide acceptance by the medical profession, to be the height of folly. I believe it puts you at great risk, and I urge you not to submit to it. If you are taking a necessary drug and you experience significant untoward side-effects, talk to your doctor and insist on a different, not an additional medication. This advice may save your life.

Nutritional supplements

What about the role of nutritional supplements in a healthy diet? No pill can substitute for eating well, for consuming a diet of whole foods which contain a complex of nutrients which work together to promote health. Nonetheless, nutritional supplements have become very popular and may be beneficial. It is beyond the scope of this book to offer advice about these supplements. I believe that you can find valuable support from a certified nutritionist who can advise you which supplements to take based on your individual history. Be aware that conventional medical doctors are not trained in nutrition.

Food

Healthy nutrition is an *individual* matter. The old aphorism, "One man's meat is another man's poison." happens to be true. Some people thrive on red meat while others feel sick after eating it. You might do well with raw fruits and vegetables while the same raw foods give your friend an upset stomach. How do you discover what are the right foods for you?

Listen to your body

Pay attention to how you are affected by what you eat. After eating, make note of foods that make you feel drowsy, bloated, nauseous, flatulent, constipated, nervous or fuzzy-headed. Your body may not digest those foods well, or you may have a food-related allergy.

Books and articles abound relating your ideal diet to your blood type or personality type or body structure. There may be some truth to all of them but for the most part you will be misled by them. Aside from the fact that many of these books contradict one another, the author of the book does not know you and reading a book can not make you an expert in his or her theory.

Let us find out if it is advisable to change the diet you are currently eating. Here are several good reasons for making changes to your food intake:

One: Suppose you are feeling fine and free of symptoms but you are consuming certain foods such as high-fructose corn syrup or trans fats that you know have been linked to serious diseases (just as you know that smoking causes lung cancer). Ask yourself why you have not stopped eating toxic items. Taking this step is not exceptionally difficult or prohibitively expensive. Read the labels and stop buying those food items that contain ingredients you know to be toxic. There are healthy substitutes for those poisons available in almost all food stores nowadays and even in most restaurants if you ask.

Two: You have heard and believe that eating fresh, whole foods in their natural state, as opposed to highly processed foods, enhances health. Why not act on this knowledge?

Three: An even more compelling reason is that you are feeling lousy and/or have specific symptoms and you suspect that may have something to do with your diet. You may not know how or where to begin to make changes. Your doctor will likely be of little or no help here. He or she will want to prescribe medication to control the symptoms you are experiencing. The drugs may even work for awhile. However, you are paying too great a price. You may develop side-effects from the medications (some of which can be dangerous) and of equal importance this approach does nothing to get at the root cause of the problem. Why not try the Elimination diet outlined in this chapter first.

Four: Or it may be that you simply wish to look or feel better, live longer and prevent disease from developing in the future. In this case, the 7 Guidelines for Eating Well presented at the conclusion of this chapter are a great place to start.

Five: Even if you are feeling lousy, it may turn out that food is not the main source of your misery. It could be your workplace that is making you sick, or perhaps stress or your own emotions are wreaking havoc on your body. Anything in your life might be affecting your health and in fact most chronic states are caused by a combination of factors. However, even if you discover that your diet is not the root cause, I would encourage you to consider following the 7 Guidelines for Eating Well for a simple reason. No matter what is what is making you sick, you can be sure that eating an unhealthy diet will make it worse.

Elimination Diet

Here is a painless, cost-free, fool proof way to determine if what you are eating is making you sick. If you are chronically or seriously ill and you suspect that what you're ingesting may be involved, consider embarking upon a more radical approach to discover which foods are problematic. You can find out whether a food allergy or irritation might be triggering or worsening your condition by eating only whole foods and eliminating gluten, dairy products, nightshades, nuts, seeds, legumes, eggs and grains for 21 days. Adding back one food at a time and noting its effects will tell you which foods are problematic for you. Even if you are not ill, trying out this "anti-inflammatory" diet (detailed in Chapter 52) periodically can make you feel great, giving your body a rest and recharging its resources to maintain health. Keep in mind that in general, the body needs about three days to fully adjust to a change in diet.

A more incremental approach involves keeping a food journal and eliminating just the foods that seem to cause problems. Every time you eat or drink, jot it down in your journal along with any positive or negative bodily response you notice. After several days or weeks you can go back through your journal and notice any patterns, positive or negative. You can also use a journal to determine if a particular food is causing a problem.

Let's say that you are experiencing weakness and fatigue and you suspect that sugar is the culprit. Take out a sheet of lined paper and down the side list the days of the week for two weeks. Across the top make categories for the things you will need to observe and record: sleep pattern, energy level, mood, bowel movements, and specific symptoms. I am not kidding about the bowel movements – they are often a very sensitive indicator of your overall health. Specific symptoms are those you have been experiencing on an ongoing basis (for example, stomach or intestinal distress, asthma or sinusitis, fatigue and weakness, and so on). You get the idea.

Next, *totally* eliminate sugar[3] or other suspect food from your diet for the next two weeks and diligently record what happens in your chart. Do not make any assumptions until the two weeks are up. If you feel better after two days of no sugar that's wonderful but keep going with the plan. At the end of the two weeks carefully study your chart and you will know if you have struck gold or not.

If your weakness and fatigue are considerably improved at the end of the test period, then it's very likely that sugar is a factor. I would not recommend that you challenge yourself by going back on sugar to see if your symptoms recur and here is why. Your body may have begun to heal enough in the two week period

---

[3] Read the label and look for sugar's key synonyms such as fructose, dextrose, sucrose, lactose (anything ending in "ose" is a sugar), any kind of syrup.

so that it would be able to 'tolerate' some sugar without developing symptoms for quite awhile. You might even delude yourself into thinking, "Oh, it wasn't the sugar after all, and the holidays are coming up and I so love Mom's Christmas cookies….." Don't do it! Be strong. Stay off sugar totally for several months and if you then want to challenge yourself with small amounts, go ahead, but keep your chart handy.

If your record keeping tells you that sugar is not the problem, you should then move on to the next category of foods that are suspect. Follow the same procedure for red meat, or wheat, or processed foods or anything else you think might be an issue. Don't forget about alcohol. I have had patients who found that their bodies could not even tolerate one or two glasses of wine with dinner.

In sum, if you find that a specific category of foods is making you sick, eliminate it from your diet right away. But your commitment to transitioning to a generally healthy diet as a preventive measure should be taken slowly; slow enough so that it does not create a stressful situation for you and your family. The 'gung-ho' approach almost always fails, and the person gives up in disgust, convincing himself that a healthy diet is nonsense. If you start by simply eliminating high-fructose corn syrup and trans fats from your diet, after a while you will find yourself craving healthy foods, making the rest of the transition much easier. One thing to keep in mind – whenever you begin eating better, you may initially feel worse as your body adjusts and/or detoxifies. For example, it is not uncommon to have headaches when giving up caffeine. Paying attention and taking your time are important principles. Wean yourself from unhealthy foods gradually and give your body at least three days to catch up to your new eating pattern.

The 7 Guidelines for Eating Well

Is it possible to eat yourself well? I believe it is, just as it is possible to eat yourself sick. We are what we eat. Whatever you swallow becomes a part of your body, so there is no better way to improve your health than to give more thought to what and how you eat. Eating well is one of the great pleasures of life. In addition to providing sustenance, eating well connects us with cultures, traditions, our families and communities. Eating well is a painless, relatively inexpensive and fun way to maintain and improve health.

So what do I mean by "eating well?" There are many different kinds of diets that humans thrive upon; however the "normal" American diet is not one of these as evidenced by the high rates of obesity, diabetes, heart disease and cancer among our population. These chronic diseases are to some extent caused by problems with what and how we eat. Fortunately it is quite easy to opt-out of this diet and its associated diseases by following the guidelines presented here.

If you are presently healthy, there is no better time to improve your diet to prevent disease and increase your healthy lifespan. After a few months of eating better you will enjoy higher energy, fewer aches and pains, a healthy shape, glowing skin, shiny hair and generally look and feel younger. If you are experiencing physical difficulty then follow the advice of Hippocrates and "Let your food be medicine and your medicine be food." This section gives you the guidelines for a healthy balanced diet, which is always the place to start.

You will find specific food suggestions for individual ailments in the relevant chapter in Part II.

Guideline 1: Eat whole foods

Our bodies are well-adapted to eating whole foods in their natural state and poorly adapted to eating highly processed foods or products of food science. Whole foods are easy to recognize, as they look like parts of the plants or animals from which they come. Ideally, the processing (e.g. cutting, slicing, dicing, mashing, cooking, seasoning) of foods we eat should take place just before we eat them. The healthfulness of food deteriorates as we increase the amount of processing and the length of time between picking, processing and eating.

Eating a well-balanced diet means about two-thirds vegetables and one-third everything else (e.g. meat, eggs, fruit, or grains). Eat as wide a variety of foods as possible and incorporate fresh raw fruit in place of processed snack foods. Your body needs fresh clean water every day to digest food, eliminate toxins and maintain balance. Drink water in between meals in place of coffee, soda or other drinks. Avoid potentially toxic and polluting plastic bottles in favor of glass or stainless steel refillable bottles.

Eating local food is a current trend. The freshness, ripeness and nutritional value of local produce is likely superior to foods shipped long distances. High quality local foods can be conveniently obtained by subscribing to a CSA (Community Supported Agriculture), where the farmer will deliver fresh produce to your door. The next best thing to CSA is shopping at your local farmer's market, where you can browse among the wares of many farmers. The produce section of your grocery store will have lots of whole foods to choose from regardless of the season. Always choose organic if it's available because organic produce will have had fewer toxins applied and will not be genetically modified. Meat and eggs should likewise be obtained from farmers, should be hormone and antibiotic-free, and be from animals that are pastured (raised naturally outside) whenever possible. These products are nutritionally better for you with higher levels of good "omega-3" fats and lower levels of toxic chemicals. Fish should be wild caught if possible for the same reasons.

Prepare your own food to the greatest extent possible. Homemade food from whole ingredients is richer in nutrients and free of preservatives, stabilizers, flavor enhancers and other toxins added to store bought food. Use all the parts of the food. Eat fruits and vegetables with their skins. Prepare stock by simmering left over vegetables (for 1 hour) or bones (for 24-48 hours) from roasted chicken, turkey, duck, pork, lamb, beef and fish, strain the liquid into containers and freeze for later use. Cook with homemade stock and its gelatin will prevent gastrointestinal infection and aid digestion. These tips will save your money and your health.

Guideline 2: Boost your body's defenses

Certain foods have a particularly strong positive effect on the body and its defenses against disease. The pigments in brightly colored fruits, vegetables and berries contain many anti-oxidant and anti-inflammatory properties. Make sure you eat the skin of these fruits and vegetables as that is where these helpful chemicals are most concentrated. Some other foods that boost the immune system are: garlic, ginger, green tea, turmeric, maitake, shiitake, and reishi mushrooms, fresh herbs like echinacea, burdock, dandelion and oregano and seaweeds such as nori, dulse, hijiki, kombu, kelp, arame and wakame.

Including more of these foods in your everyday diet will improve your health and help you avoid disease.

Guideline 3: Choose healthy fats

Despite the ubiquitous rhetoric about "low fat" diets, eating a certain amount of fat is essential for your health. Healthy fats include coconut oil, butter, olive oil and fats in naturally raised food (fish, meat, poultry, seeds and nuts). Eating these foods helps reduce inflammation and can help prevent premature aging and many diseases. Foods high in omega-3 essential fatty acids have a very powerful anti-inflammatory effect. These include cold water oily fish (particularly wild salmon), walnuts, flax seeds, and pumpkin seeds. Extra virgin olive oil and natural coconut oil will also reduce inflammation and reduce the risk of heart disease.

Guideline 4: Stop eating junk

Junk food is not food. Junk foods include sweeteners, processed meats, unhealthy fats and additives which will increase inflammation in your body. Eliminating this non-food from your diet is just as important as incorporating healthy whole foods. Anything that is so highly processed as to be potentially harmful to your health, or that contributes calories without nutrition is junk. To improve your health and longevity eliminate the following:

Sweet-tasting drinks (e.g. soda, diet soda, energy drinks, sports drinks) – the artificial sweeteners and/or sugars in these drinks cause a host of problems. Nutrasweet and high fructose corn syrup are two of the worst culprits. Even juice drinks have too much concentrated sugar for the body to absorb all at once. Drink plenty of water instead.

Salty packaged snacks (e.g. chips, crisps, puffs, popcorn, crackers) – these snacks pack an unhealthy dose of salt and may also contain toxic trans fats (partially hydrogenated oils), artificial flavors and colors. Snack on fresh fruits or vegetables instead. Try raw nuts for variety (soak them in water the night before).

Fast food and convenience food – Most people realize that whatever you buy at a drive-through window is going to be nutritionally poor quality. Not as many people realize that the same is true of anything that goes from your freezer to your microwave oven. If you're in a hurry at home, eat a salad with vegetables, fruit, nuts or a hard-boiled egg and home-made salad dressing. Instead of a fast-food drive through, drop into a deli or the prepared foods section of a grocery store and get a fresh sandwich or soup and salad to go.

There are other easy ways to identify non-food. For example, if it never spoils (e.g. Twinkies, Gummi Bears and other packaged sweets) it's not food. If you are buying it at a gas station, it's probably not food and it's certainly not good food. If high fructose corn syrup is an ingredient, then it's probably not food. If the ingredients list has anything in it you can't recognize (monoglycerides?) then it's probably not food.

Guideline 5: Make it a treat

If there are certain things you enjoy very much - make them a special treat. If you eat chocolate cake every day you will enjoy it less and the spiking of your blood sugar will take a toll on your health. If you make chocolate cake an occasional treat you will enjoy anticipating and eating it much more and the health effects will be negligible. You can apply this principle to any guilty pleasure such as drinking coffee or alcohol. If you find it impossible to make these things a treat, then moderation is the next best thing.

Guideline 6: Avoid anti-nutrients through soaking and cooking

I've heard it said that the healthiest diet is to eat only raw food. Not so! Some raw foods naturally contain anti-nutrients and toxins. Fortunately, these are easily dispersed or destroyed by soaking and/or cooking.

Nuts and seeds should be soaked overnight in clean spring, well or filtered water at room temperature. After soaking, discard the water and use the nuts in recipes as you normally would. You will find them softened and more delicious than before soaking. Dehydrating or lightly roasting soaked nuts and seeds is fine, but take care not to overcook and use up each batch within a few days.

Foods that may be less healthful eaten raw include:

- Legumes and pulses (e.g. alfalfa, clover, peas, beans, lentils, lupins, mesquite, carob, soy and peanuts). Soaking and sprouting helps significantly, although some people may still have difficulty with alfalfa sprouts.
- Cruciferous vegetables (e.g. arugula, broccoli, kale, cauliflower, cabbage, turnip, collard greens, bok choy, brussels sprouts, radish, rutabaga, and watercress) as well as spinach, chard, parsely, chives, purslane and beet greens. Lightly steam

or boil these in water and discard the water. Sautéing or roasting are also fine.

- Potatoes and sweet potatoes should not be eaten raw, and you must remove any blemishes, wounds, sprouts or eyes before cooking.
- Red cabbage
- Button or Portobello mushrooms (as a rule I don't eat any mushroom raw)
- Cassava (contains toxins and should not be eaten raw).
- Nightshade vegetables (potatoes, tomatoes, sweet and hot peppers, eggplant, tomatillos, tamarios, pepinos, pimentos, paprika, cayenne). Tabasco sauce is also classified as a nightshade food. Cooking reduces the problems associated with these foods, but individuals who are sensitive to them may not be able to eat them even when cooked. I find fresh tomatoes delightful, but pay attention to make sure you do not have any negative reaction to eating them raw.

If you must eat any of these foods raw, do so in small quantities. It may be more work to wilt or sauté your spinach salad, but it's better than developing kidney stones, isn't it?

Guideline 7: Pay attention

It's almost impossible to pay attention to what you're eating and how it affects you these days. Music, noise, television and conversation make it very difficult to eat consciously. When you eat, do you feel as though you are "dining" or "refueling?" Whenever possible, just eat – doing nothing else but enjoying the meal.

Simply paying attention to the meal can greatly enhance your pleasure as well as your health.

Pay attention to how your body reacts to foods and listen to your body's wisdom. If you take a bite of fish and your mouth starts to itch, spit it out and avoid a painful case of food poisoning. Likewise if something you eat causes an adverse reaction later on, find out what it is and stop eating it. This may seem so obvious as to be useless advice, but in fact, most people go on eating things that affect them negatively, oblivious to the fact that their health is being ruined by something completely within their control to avoid.

It takes some time for your body to signal that it is full. If you eat too fast, you will have consumed a great deal more than you need before you notice these signals. Here is a great way to slow down: take a bite of food and put your fork or spoon down while you chew and swallow that one bite completely before picking up your fork or spoon again. Constantly fishing for the next bite while chewing leads to a "shoveling" form of eating which is bound to result in eating too much. Eating slowly will also allow you to really taste and enjoy each bite.

At its best, dining can be a blissful meditation and celebration as you take nourishment from food. Food prepared with love and eaten with consciousness engenders those qualities in you and enhances your health and well-being.

4 THE SECOND PILLAR - EXERCISE

The sovereign invigorator of the body is exercise, and of all exercises walking is the best.
- Thomas Jefferson

You may be tempted to skip over this chapter because, after all, everyone knows that exercise is necessary to good health and most everyone knows what constitutes a good exercise program. These assumptions warrant closer examination.

"Exercise." The first thing that comes to most people's minds is some form of vigorous 'aerobic' movement: competitive sports, workouts at the gym, running or jogging or speed walking, biking, hiking, and so forth. In recent years, getting fit or 'ripped' seems to be a sine qua non for our very survival. I have noticed that even the 5000 year old practice of yoga has moved in the direction of a power workout. Hot yoga, indeed!

I have no quarrel with vigorous, heart-rate-elevating, sweat-breaking exercise. Especially if you are young and your work and home life are stress-filled, go for it. It's a great escape, it will enhance your cardio-respiratory function, and it's a far better way to socialize than hanging out in bars.

But as you get older, say beyond thirty-something, be careful to avoid the effects of repetitive trauma on your joints or you may be rendered unable to exercise at all. Think again before taking anti-inflammatory drugs to relieve the aches and pains associated with your work-outs. Pain is like a friend grabbing you by the arm when you are about to step out into oncoming traffic. Pay attention to what your body is trying to tell you. If you are hurting, take a break, or short rests, or cut back on your program until you are free of pain.

As you move into your forties and beyond, consider this. There is no evidence that high-powered exercises will enhance your health or longevity any more than two miles of energetic walking each day. Seriously, the benefits of power workouts over walking are largely cosmetic and ego-boosting. You may consider walking to be mundane and unexciting and it is often a solitary pursuit, but for health enhancement, it can't be beat. It can also be used as a meditation, as we will see later in the book.

If you do choose to walk, I offer the following advice. Aim for a speed of about three miles per hour. If possible, walk in nature on soft surfaces such as grass or gravel and seek out hilly terrain. If cement roads or sidewalks are all that is available to you, then be sure to wear good quality walking shoes to protect yourself from repetitive jarring injury. Here is another helpful hint if walking on a hard surface. Every quarter mile or so walk backwards for a few yards, then skip sideways awhile, or in some other way change your stride.

Most people are unaware that there are several other categories of exercise that are even more effective than aerobics in achieving optimal health and well-being. These varieties of exercise become especially important as you move beyond middle age and are, in my opinion, essential if your health is already compromised in some way.

They can be roughly divided into the following types:

- Breath and Voice Exercises
- Flexibility Exercises
- Expressive Exercises
- Mental/Brain Exercises
- Sexual Exercises

As we will see, the distinctions are somewhat artificial, as many of the techniques overlap each other. For example, we use the voice in expressive exercise as well as the body. In fact, all of these are Mind/Body exercises. In the remainder of this chapter we will define each of these categories, give examples, and discuss how and why they are helpful in health promotion and disease prevention. Most of these exercises are relatively easy to perform. The biggest stumbling block you will face is mild embarrassment at doing something that others might consider 'weird.' But then, you are already reading this book.

Breath and Voice Exercises

The first thing everyone does coming into the world is to take the breath of life. The last thing we do on this earth is expire. Watch an infant breathe. See the belly rise with each inhalation and fall as he breathes out. It is a free, easy and unconscious process.

Most adults do not breathe freely and easily, even those who do not have a respiratory condition. Starting in childhood and continuing through our formative years, we unconsciously restrict our breathing in order to meet the demands of everyday life. In addition we may habitually hold in the stomach in an attempt to uphold an expectation of body shape all the while restricting our flow of breath.

When we are physically exerting ourselves, there is a normal impulse to groan or shout at times with the effort, but we have learned not to do that. Most of us (especially men) think it is not socially acceptable. Instead we tend to hold our breaths, as if that would be helpful. Even more common is the unconscious restriction of our breathing when we begin to experience strong emotion. We are afraid of being seen as inappropriate if we shout or scream or cry or even laugh at times. This holding back, or inhibition, of the breath is an automatic process; we are unaware that we are doing it.

The more severe the restriction, the more likely we are to develop diseases and conditions as a result of the long-standing inhibition of full, free and easy respiration. And the problems are not limited to the lungs. In addition to asthma, chronic obstructive pulmonary disease (COPD), and frequent respiratory infections, we are at risk for digestive disorders (especially gastro-esophageal reflux disorder, also known as GERD), heart disease and anxiety. Sounds far-fetched? Not at all. Notice that I did not say that restricted breathing causes these conditions. But it does pre-dispose us to them. And learning to open our breathing, to make it full and free and easy, can reverse the predisposition and in my experience with patients, it is sometimes all that is required to get better.

There is an infinite variety of useful breath and voice exercises, coming from different healing traditions. Some of them are detailed in Part II under specific diseases and conditions. In addition, the ones that I have found most useful are detailed in Chapter 45. But right now, before reading further, try this simple observation to determine if your breathing pattern needs work.

Lie on your back with a small pillow under your neck. Bend your legs at the knees so that your feet rest flat on the floor. Place a fairly large book on your abdomen, right over your navel. Breathe normally for a few breaths, then take in a large breath. Really fill your lungs with air. Hold if for a moment, then let it go, slowly.

Did the book rise as you took the big breath in? Or did the book not move, or did it perhaps even move lower with your inhalation? If the book did not rise with inhalation and fall with exhalation (like the infant breath noted above) then your breathing is restricted and you will especially benefit from the breath and voice exercises.

The restriction of our respiration comes about as a result of chronic muscular tension in our throat, chest, belly and most of all, our diaphragm. I wish to emphasize that this tension occurs without our conscious knowledge. But we can use our conscious minds, our will, to correct the problem by doing the breathing exercises and learning to become aware of tension and of ways to let it go. Even if you do not have any of the diseases associated with restricted breathing, learning and practicing some of the breath and voice techniques will enhance your overall health as you age.

Flexibility Exercises

Young children move with ease and grace. They can get themselves into postures that would be the envy of advanced yoga practitioners. In later childhood, we learn to restrict our movements for much the same reasons I mentioned above in the section on Breath. Over the years, without our awareness, we develop chronic tensions in our skeletal muscles, in the areas of our limbs or trunk or head and neck. This chronic muscular tension predisposes us to actual disease states over time.

Tension in the head and neck can result in headaches and temporal mandibular joint disorder (TMJ). Tension in the back can lead to scoliosis, lordosis, and acute and chronic back pain. In the pelvis, sexual difficulties and problems related to bowel and bladder. In the legs, knee, hip and ankle problems. Certain forms of arthritis, as we shall see, are linked to chronic tension in the muscles surrounding the joints.

Strength training and certain sports do nothing to enhance flexibility and may in fact result in more chronic muscular tension. If you are involved in these pursuits, it would serve you well to do flexibility training as well.

Certainly the most popular and potentially most effective form of flexibility training is yoga. Yoga can be a life-changing and health enhancing practice, especially if done on a daily basis.

A really good yoga class will not only enhance your flexibility but will also incorporate breathing and energizing exercises as well. To teach all of this well, the instructor needs years of training and experience and to some extent the wisdom that comes with age. And, equally important, he or she needs to be able to individualize the process, to be able to see the 'energetic flow' (or lack of it) in each person and to know how to correct it with words or touch. If you have heard about such a teacher in your area, sign up right away.

There are other varieties of flexibility training and/or techniques to enhance freedom of movement and correct postural alignment. Some of these include tai chi, Alexander technique, Feldenkreis and nia. Again, the most important factor is the skill of the instructor. Try to find some information on the training and experience of the teacher before signing up. Perhaps you can observe or participate in a class before signing up for a series. Notice whether the teacher is able to respond to the individual needs of each student. If you feel uncomfortable or unsafe in a class, ask the advice of the teacher. If this advice leaves you unsatisfied, try another teacher.

What about learning yoga and related disciplines from a DVD? I do not recommend this unless you are an experienced practitioner and wish to learn advanced techniques at home. One of the many benefits a teacher can offer is feedback on the correct way to perform each movement for maximum benefit.

In Part II of this book, under specific diseases and conditions, you will find certain exercises to enhance flexibility that are usually linked to enhancing energetic flow in the body. Most of these are derived from Bioenergetics, a discipline which I studied extensively and have been practicing for decades. I believe you will find them most helpful and a pleasure to perform. I encourage you to try them out and see for yourself.

Expressive Exercises

What do I mean by expressive exercises? Some of you may have heard about laughter classes that are especially popular in India. Those of you who are older will recall 'getting your yah-yahs out' from the 1970's, or groups where people pound pillows and scream. If you are reading this and are already getting nervous or turned off, then this category is probably just what you need.

I want to make a very strong statement here. *The free flow of energy and feeling through the body is the most effective deterrent to the development of chronic disease states.*

I am not referring here to 'acting-out.' You do not have to dump on others, either verbally or physically, in order to feel better. In fact, in the long run, that behavior will make you feel worse. I am talking about allowing ourselves to experience the full gamut of our emotions.

Hopefully, most of you have had the experience of wild, nearly uncontrollable laughter in certain social situations. Do you recall a sense of aliveness and joy immediately afterwards? Or perhaps you recall a time when you had a 'really good cry,' and felt cleansed and happy for awhile. In order to have a good laugh or a good cry, we have to let down our defenses, which literally means relaxing our muscular armoring, if only briefly. Then our energy and our feelings can flow freely, some might say our cells are happy, and at those moments we are in a state of optimal health.

Note that I have linked energy and feeling in this category. We can certainly raise our energy level without stirring up our feelings. For example, by doing some of the exercises we have already mentioned, such as aerobic training and a good yoga class. Raising our energy level does not mean that energy is flowing freely through our bodies. Check yourself out the next time you engage in strenuous exercise. Is there a frown on your face, is your jaw tight, are your shoulders tense, is your belly rigid, do you feel tension in your legs? If you notice these and/or other areas of tension, then your energy is not flowing freely. You have unconsciously blocked the flow by tightening the muscles. You are doing this because it is an old habit. In order to 'perform' well many of us think we need to concentrate hard and squeeze out our best effort. And we need to keep our mouths shut while we are doing it and express neither our misery (moans and groans) or our joy (hoots and hollers) in the situation.

This holding back is a cultural expectation in "polite society." In other cultures, open expression of feeling is more acceptable in social situations and the workplace. I suspect that people in those cultures lead happier and healthier lives.

Most young children are energetic and expressive. I worry about the ones who are not. Watch a little girl who is excited about something – a visit to the amusement park or a ride on daddy's shoulders – and you will see what I mean about the full flow of energy and feeling. Her eyes are bright, the skin is flushed, she might jump up and down and clap her hands and squeal or laugh with delight.

A few people I know retain that 'flow' into adulthood. Although they no longer jump for joy when excited, you can still see the sparkle in their eyes and a healthy glow on their cheeks and watch them grin from ear to ear or even laugh aloud and rub their hands together in anticipation. I do not worry about the health of these lucky people.

Isn't it odd that most of us hold back even our excitement, which is a perfectly acceptable emotion to show to the world. The reason is that when we are taught as young children that certain of our emotions are not acceptable (such as anger or sadness) we shut down these feelings by constricting our musculature. When this becomes a chronic state, then the expression of *all* feeling is inhibited. I want to emphasize again that this is not a choice we are making. It is an unconscious process.

We can not *will* ourselves to start opening to the flow of energy and feeling through our bodies. If we have been shut down for years, the 'channels' have to be opened slowly, and you can learn safe and effective exercises from this book that will do just that. However, you have to *want* that to happen. You may want to improve your health, but you may not be willing to risk experiencing those emotions that have been shut down for so long. You must first make a conscious choice...the choice toward growth and change.

We would like to be able to be selective about our feelings. You might be thinking, well, happiness and perhaps even sadness are acceptable, but anger is not. You might even convince yourself (perhaps influenced by new-age slogans) that anger is bad for your health – you've heard it called a negative emotion – and bad for the planet as well. But there are no negative emotions. Feelings are feelings are feelings. And before you draw unwarranted conclusions about that, let me hasten to add: while we must *experience* our feelings in order to achieve good health, we do not have to *act* on them.

So let us look at 'seething.' I choose that word because I'm sure you have all experienced that at some point. One could easily include the feeling states of resentment and hostility in this category. I have often asked a patient how they felt in such and such a situation when things did not go their way. "Oh, I was seething." I respond by reminding them that seething is not an emotion. It is an unpleasant physical response to holding back a feeling, usually anger. "Well," they ask, "what did you want me to do, get up and punch the guy in the face or scream at him?"

Here the patient is making the classic mistake of assuming that if he allows the feeling of anger to flow freely through his body, then he must act it out. *Seething feels awful and doesn't go away quickly. Anger feels good and dissipates quickly.* You may understand this, but you will not know what I mean until you have experienced it for yourself. Expressive exercises can give you that somatic knowledge (knowing it in your body).

Still you have doubts. I hear you saying, 'I have experienced anger and it did not feel good. I felt very tense and like I was going to explode.' Yes, I'm sure you were angry, but what you were experiencing in your body was seething or even perhaps suppressed rage. In either case, you were contracted.

When we are angry in a healthy adult way, we expand: we appear larger, flushed, breathing fully and freely and we feel very alive. We may have the desire to punch out somebody and can feel that impulse in our arms and fists. We also have the impulse to roar, like a lion, as we attack. In my practice, I teach patients how to feel their anger and respond in an appropriate, non-damaging way. Rather than acting out the impulses, we can look our 'opponent' (who at this point might be our beloved spouse or a valued co-worker) in the eyes and say something like, 'that really makes me angry' or

'I just do not feel heard or understood.' We tell the other person what we are experiencing. Period. We stay in contact with them and wait for a response.

I have stressed that we need to stay in contact with the other person. This is very important. It marks the difference between anger and rage. Hence the expressions 'blind rage' or 'mindless rage.' Rage is an infantile response to NOT being in contact with the other. You will not witness a child having a temper tantrum and looking you in the eye at the same time. When we are enraged we disconnect from our adult selves and from the person with whom we are angry. If you really *see* the other person and keep in mind who he or she is, you will not experience rage.

What does all this have to do with our health? Everything. There is so much misinformation out there about our feelings. But the facts are simple. We are human, therefore we feel. If we allow our emotions to flow through our bodies, they will subside quickly and our health we be enhanced. If we contract against them, especially if this becomes a chronic process, our health is compromised.

If you are a person who 'seeths' and cannot let go of the tension associated with that phenomenon, I urge you to try some of the expressive exercises in Chapter 47. They are safe and sane and are necessary for most of us in our present day culture. And, if you do not judge them or yourself, you may even find them to be fun.

In our culture it is not acceptable for adults to cry openly except in exceptional circumstances such as death of a loved one or the destruction of our home by fire or flood. Noisy crying and sobbing makes other people nervous. They may try to comfort us by resurrecting what they heard as children, saying 'everything is OK, don't cry.' How silly. Of course everything is not OK. Crying is a natural phenomenon that is an expression of deep sadness and loss. And it is very cleansing.

When we suppress our crying or are unaware that we need to cry, we set ourselves up for stagnation of energy flow which in turn can lead to disease. I am convinced that behind most cases of recurrent and chronic sinusitis is the need to cry, fully and openly. It can be even more pervasive than that. I would like to share something from my own medical history to illustrate what I mean.

Galen was a Shepard-Lab mix, the first dog I owned as an adult. I got him as a puppy shortly after moving to the farm. He was my constant companion for nine years. One day he began acting sick and refused to eat. After two more days I took him to our vet who, after examining him, told me that his abdomen was filled with cancer. To end his suffering, I had him put down right then and there, on the floor of the office, with me holding his head in my lap. I cried for a few moments, then pulled myself together and went to work.

A week later I came down with a strange illness. I felt totally drained, weak and was unable to eat anything. By the next day I was too weak to get out of bed for longer than a few minutes. I had no fever and no specific symptoms except a dull ache in my solar plexus. One of my doctor friends examined me and found nothing remarkable. He suggested hospitalization for tests if I did not improve in a couple of days. By the fifth day I was convinced I had a fatal illness.

In despair I called my best friend and told him what I was going through. This friend is not a doctor but he is very perceptive and he knows me like a book. He asked me what had been going on in my life recently. I had not told him, or anyone else outside the family, about the loss of my beloved dog.

I tried to tell him about Galen's death, but I was choking on the words. Finally I simply blurted out "Galen died," and began to sob uncontrollably. He wisely said nothing except perhaps uh-huh, softly. Finally I was able to say, between more sobs, "I miss him so much." We exchanged a few more words and I suddenly realized I was hungry. I got out of bed and ate. Within a couple of hours my strength and energy were back and I was able to resume normal activities.

I believe that I might have died if I had not been able to express my grief. Oh, not right away. I would have gone to the hospital, gotten re-hydrated with intravenous feedings and sent home. Probably I would have been up and down for awhile and eventually I would have been diagnosed with cancer or some awful 'auto-immune' disease, treated with toxic medications and would ultimately succumb to the disease without anyone ever knowing what caused it.

Some of you reading this may know that you need to cry, but can't. In Chapter 47 there are specific suggestions for ways to facilitate that process.

Mental/Brain Exercises

This category is intended primarily for those of us who have progressed beyond middle age and have not as yet been labeled by the medical profession as demented. Perhaps you are forgetful or 'absent-minded' or a bit 'dotty' but are still a functioning member of society. If so, these remarks are for you (and me).

Prevention. Prevention. Prevention. It can not be said often enough. There is not a lot you can do once you have lost brain cells, but so much can be done to prevent the loss. In addition to good nutrition (perhaps with certain supplements) and an age-appropriate exercise program, certain mind/brain exercises can be very useful.

Most of this is self-evident. First, stop watching so much TV. Don't rely on your computer for spell-checking – look it up. Balance your checkbook manually, without a calculator. Do crossword puzzles. Learn a foreign language.

I have found meditation to be particularly useful in this regard. You are never too old to learn meditation. In fact, I have found that older folks take to it much more readily than their younger counterparts. Perhaps it is simply that we are willing to make time for it in our lives. It can lead us to great mental clarity when done properly. This will be discussed at great length in Chapter 5. In addition, there are a couple of very specific 'active meditations' which can be done to enhance cognitive functioning. These are detailed in Chapter 48.

Sexual Exercises

Like other feelings, the free flow of sexual energy is important for our health and well-being. How can we know if our sexual arousal, masturbation and intercourse are health-enhancing activities and not simply a distraction from our daily grind and a release of pent-up tension? Self-awareness and close observation will provide the answer.

In general, if you feel happy and energized for several hours after sexual activity, it is good for your health. But if you are a person who feels depleted, empty and 'down' after sex, you may be doing yourself more harm than good. Please do not jump to the conclusion that I am suggesting that you need to curtail your sex life. You need a fresh approach to your sexual activity to make it more health enhancing and this book will provide you with the tools to do just that.

It is useful to observe the pattern of our sexual arousal. Some of us become aroused through thoughts and visual images about sex. Others do so by self-stimulation or the touch of another. Still others need intimate emotional contact with a significant other. A lucky few become aroused simply by feeling alive and energized. All of this is normal. There is no 'right' way.

Once your arousal begins, notice where if goes. If it is strictly a genital sensation, you are missing out on a lot. Ideally, as the level of arousal mounts, it is felt throughout the body: breathing becomes deeper and faster; the skin, especially along the front of the body, becomes flushed and tingly; your mouth craves contact; and your pelvis begins to move spontaneously. At this point, if your only objective is release – ejaculation for men, orgasm for women – you are robbing yourself of some exquisite (and health-enhancing) pleasure.

Especially if you have reached middle-age, don't rush to release, regardless of how much pleasure it brings you. Cultivate the full-body sensation of arousal. You might even consider (especially if you are a man) forgoing release on some occasions and letting the 'glow' of sex stay with you all day. This is the best form of sexual exercise. You might even find that you don't need that boring 'work-out' at the gym.

A number of you, especially those beyond middle-age, may be experiencing a lack of sexual desire. It carries many labels: impotence, frigidity, erectile dysfunction, loss of libido. Regardless of your diagnosis, most of you can regain sexual arousal by the natural means detailed in this chapter and in Part III.

But let us first look at the main causes of lack of sexual desire. These are generally thought to be fatigue, 'stress,' unhappy relationships, excessive alcohol intake, smoking, overwork and unresolved issues around sexual abuse. All of these are very important and need to be dealt with. However, in my opinion, the single most common cause of lack of libido is medications, prescription and/or over the counter drugs. I have no proof that this is the case, but it has been my personal and clinical experience that it is an accurate observation. If you agree that this is an important factor for you, but feel hopeless because you need your meds, take heart. If you enhance your health by following the natural methods outlined in this book, you will be able to reduce or eliminate most of your medications, and will hopefully experience a return of your sexual desire and functioning.

A word of caution to those of you who may be tempted to take one of the widely advertised drugs for erectile dysfunction: As is the case for most of the commonly prescribed medications on the market today, the dangers and side-effects of these drugs are given in very small print, or in the case of TV advertising, the hazards are mentioned *sotto voce*, as if they didn't matter. Pay attention to these warnings and then think about whether you still want to take these drugs. And consider this. Do you honestly believe that an oral medication powerful enough to give you an erection, can NOT have effects on the rest of your body? How do you think it gets to your penis? It is absorbed in your intestine and circulates through your bloodstream, available to every organ in your body. What are you risking here? Nobody knows, yet.

If you are able to discontinue most of the medications that might be affecting your libido and you have dealt with stress and fatigue and the other issues mentioned above, and still your arousal does not return, please try the specific exercises detailed in the chapter on Impotence in Part II and see the additional exercises in Chapter 49. These exercises, by the way, do not require the participation of a sexual partner.

5 THE THIRD PILLAR – GOING TO THE SOURCE

Who had put wisdom in the inward parts?
Or who hath given understanding to the heart?
- Job 38:36
Attachment is the great fabricator of illusions;
reality can be attained only by someone who is
detached.
- Simone Weil

What do we mean by 'going to the source,' the third of the three pillars that provide the foundation for a healthy life? To me it means going to that place of stillness that is present deep within each of us. For some, this has religious connotations, perhaps of prayer. If your faith and your prayers are a source of healing for you, you may not need the advice and instruction provided in this section. For many of us, however, it will be useful to learn a technique to access this place of stillness and healing. I use the word meditation to describe this process.

Take a moment right now and try this experiment. Put the book down but stay seated in your chair. Close your eyes and picture, in your mind's eye, a place where you have always felt safe and content. Try to imagine yourself there now, on the beach or in the garden or perhaps in your grandmother's lap, and stay with that image for two or three minutes. Then open your eyes slowly and pay attention to what you are feeling in your body.

Most people are able to find a place of contentment and many are able to feel the sense of relaxation and safety that comes with this visual exercise. If this is true for you, then you may not need to do anything beyond practicing this exercise two or three times a day, perhaps for longer periods. This will provide you with the 'third pillar' - a safe haven from the stresses of daily life and in fact an antidote to the negative physiologic effects of those stresses.

How strange it is that so few people are willing to take the ten to fifteen minutes per day to restore themselves in this way. I hear all kinds of reasons: I couldn't find the time, nobody would leave me alone, I forgot, and so forth. I wonder if the real reason is a cultural one. We have grown so accustomed to a frenetic life-style that it feels normal to us, while taking a few moments to do essentially nothing may feel like a 'waste of time.' If we are to find contentment in our lives and wish to move towards optimal health, it will be necessary to get past that cultural barrier. We will have to learn to view the meditative experience as a normal and necessary part of our daily lives.

Children used to spend some time each day doing what we might now call 'zoning out.' This is a negative labeling of something that is a perfectly normal phenomenon, namely daydreaming. Daydreaming is a creative act as well as a restorative one and kids should not be discouraged from its pursuit. Of course if the TV is on all day and/or there is constant input from other electronic devices and there is a tight schedule of homework, lessons, sports and theme birthday parties, children will not have the time to do what comes naturally. They will miss out on a valuable self-healing experience and be the worse off for it. Daydreaming is the childhood version of meditation.

If you were able to find contentment from the visualization exercise and you wish to go beyond that to even more health-enhancing techniques, you will find plenty of helpful information in this section and in Chapter 50.

If you were unable to imagine a safe place or if the experiment did not work for you, please don't despair. There are many possible reasons for this and there are other ways to deal with the stresses in your life. Some of you may not be very 'visual.' You may be more auditory or even kinesthetic. In this book you will find meditative exercises that employ sound as well as finger movements that are relaxing and restorative. There is even a walking meditation.

You may ask, "Why can't I just sit and relax, listen to music, read a book or even watch TV?" Why isn't that enough to deal with stress? Here's why. Lots of clinical research has been done on the techniques of relaxation and meditation. Scientists have measured many aspects of bodily functioning during these states, such as heart rate, respiratory rate, blood pressure and brain waves, as well as the levels of stress hormones in the blood and other parameters of immune function. They found that only the meditative state provides the kind of physiologic response necessary to serve as an antidote to the ravages of stress. Even sleep, as necessary as it is to good health, does not serve the same purpose.

It is good to sit and relax by listening to music, reading a book, perhaps even watching certain programs on television. If these still moments are balanced by periods of exercise, as we have outlined previously, and if you are paying attention to your 'intake,' you are moving in the direction of good health. And if you have no current symptoms and do not experience your daily activities as particularly stressful, you might have no need for a meditative exercise. But then you probably wouldn't be reading this book.

In order for meditation to be useful to you in your quest for disease-prevention and health-promotion, those few minutes must become part of your daily routine for the rest of your life. However, you do not have to go to an ashram or attend weekend retreats. You do not have to sit in quiet rigidity for an hour, or longer. It is not even necessary for you to be seeking spiritual growth in order to gain the health benefits of meditation. In my experience, spiritual growth will come about naturally if you practice meditation on a regular basis – you will hardly notice the change, but others will. I will go even further. Those who go about extolling their spiritual path often miss out on the health benefits. Maybe they are trying too hard and thus adding stress to their lives.

Let us say that you have made the commitment and found the time to practice 'going to the source' on a daily basis. Great. You may be feeling better already. Lots of people who learn meditation from a book or CD or in a yoga class find it relaxing and pleasurable. So why do most of them give up the practice after a few weeks? The answer can be summed up in one word: Expectations.

Abandon your expectations. If you can truly do this and instead become a non-judgmental observer of what is actually happening, you will learn more about yourself than you ever dreamed possible. And self-knowledge, self-awareness, is the greatest therapeutic tool you can possess. It will lead you to the correct decisions about your health and well-being.

You may find after a few weeks that your meditation is no longer the pleasurable experience it was initially. Physical discomforts may crop up. Unpleasant emotions may surface. And, most commonly, you can not stop the incessant chatter of your mind. If any or all of these are happening, you will be tempted to stop the practice. If you do, you will be missing a great opportunity for self-awareness and growth.

You are probably thinking, how can a meditation filled with discomforts be helpful to my health? Isn't it just adding stress to my life? So what if I learn a lot about what I am thinking and feeling, that's not going to help me now.

Try this experiment, which requires an assistant. Sit in a straight-backed chair and close your eyes. Have your friend stand behind you and pinch both of your shoulders hard enough so that it really hurts you. Have him maintain that pressure while you sit quietly and give the pain your full attention. Breathe into the pain, notice it more and more each time you breathe out. Become *fully occupied* with the awareness of that pain. Please do not read beyond this paragraph until you try this experiment. Just notice what your experience is before I tell you what happens to most people.

If you were able to give the pain your full attention – not *think* about it but simply be fully present with the pain – you probably noticed that the pain diminished in intensity, perhaps even to the extent that it was barely noticeable. If so, this will have been your first lesson in Detachment. A friend puts it this way, "I first experienced the value of meditation when I meditated while I had a headache and concentrated on that pain. I learned that this was the best way to deal with headaches, and after a few months never had another headache."

Almost nothing is as bad as you think it is. Obviously I am not talking here about the horrors of war or other extreme violent acts. But in the course of our everyday lives, the 'pain' is worse because of how we think and feel about it. Learning detachment in no way means becoming an unthinking, unfeeling, uncaring person. It enables us to think more clearly and feel more deeply.

But let us get back to the discomforts that may arise during your practice of meditation. Here are some commonly experienced minor physical problems and what to do about them. Itchy skin: scratch gently as often as necessary. Aching in neck, shoulder or back: tighten, and then relax those muscles. Jumpy feet or legs: wiggle your toes. There are probably others, but you get the idea. What is happening here is that when you sit quietly and 'go inside,' you become aware of the things that have escaped your notice in your everyday state of consciousness.

Here is a bigger problem: sleepiness. Again, in your state of busy-ness you have been unaware of how tired you are. The remedy: take a short nap instead of struggling to continue the meditation.

Some people find that when they go inside powerful feelings rise to the surface. This may be preceded by nausea. Nausea during meditation is almost always a sign that a strong feeling is coming up in you while your body is doing its best to contain it. See if you can create an opening in your body for these emotions to surface. If you realize that you will not be overwhelmed by feelings, you may feel safe enough to allow this to happen. Simply continue sitting and observing as these feelings flow through you. For example, you may start crying. Good, let the tears and the sobbing happen and at the same time continue sitting still and observing, almost as if these emotions were happening to someone else. You do NOT need to understand why you are having that particular emotion, nor do you need to do anything about it.

Whatever feelings arise during meditation, handle them in the same manner. You will probably find that they subside spontaneously as you continue your sitting. If, however, strong feelings persist during your state of 'normal' consciousness for more than a day or two, then discontinue the practice and seek help from a therapist. You will be OK. It is just that the going inside practice has triggered something deep in you that needs attending to. The good news is that as you resolve the issues with the therapist, they will no longer pose a threat to your health. That is to say, you will have prevented the development of a chronic health problem.

The most common complaint I hear from people who are attempting to establish a regular practice of meditation is, "I can't seem to quiet my mind." To them I say, "neither can I." Here again the problem is one of expectations. When I teach meditation I never tell my students or patients to quiet the mind. It is a recipe for failure. And yet they keep trying, perhaps because of the common misconception that a quiet mind is necessary for meditation or healing. This is not true.

What is true is this. You have to learn to be OK with your 'chattering monkey' mind. You have to find a way to let it not be a bother to you. The secret is in coming to the realization that YOUR MIND IS NOT YOU. It would not bother you much during your meditative practice if there were noisy children playing in the street outside your window, or a flock of chirping birds around your feeder. That is the way you should view your busy mind: this is not me. I am sitting here on my chair, breathing and meditating, while my mind is running off at the mouth. Well, let it. You just go on with what you are doing. Oh, you will continue to hear the chattering, but it will become, like the monkeys in the tree, a minor annoyance to your contentment.

You will notice that with all this talk about meditation I have not taught you how to do it. The reason is that it is not a 'one size fits all' situation. One of the main reasons that so few people continue is that meditation needs to be individualized to suit the individual's life-style and personality.

There are many varieties of meditation coming from a number of ancient and not so ancient traditions. Unless you are contemplating a contemplative life, it is not fair to ask you to follow the exact practice of a specific tradition. You need to develop a practice that works for you.

There are several variables that need to be addressed such as location, time of day, posture, length of sitting, induction technique, focus, and managing 'problems' that arise. For now, what I will do is introduce you to a simple technique developed by one of my mentors. Please begin the practice and pay attention to your reactions and responses.

Location: any place where you can sit and not be disturbed by people or telephones. Can't find such a place in your home? Then it might need to be in your car, in the far reaches of a parking lot.

Time of day: almost any time except right after eating. The best times for most people seem to be morning before going to work and/or evening before dinner. Try to meditate at least once a day; twice is better.

Posture: This is very important for reasons that are not quite clear, but experience teaches that the results are best if a certain posture is followed. Find a straight-backed chair, with no 'slouch' to it. If the surface is too hard, place a thin pillow between you and the chair back or seat. Place your feet on the floor, uncrossed. Place your hands either on your thighs or folded in your lap (do not interlace the fingers). Keep your head level, chin neither down on your chest or up in the air.

Getting started: Close your eyes (but if this makes you nervous, direct your eyes to a spot on the floor some distance from your chair). Breathe out fully three times, and then begin to pay attention to your breathing, to the flow of air as it comes in and out of your body. Focus on the out-breath, the exhalation. Each time you feel your breath flowing out, *mentally* say the word ONE. Do not count the breaths, simply accompany each exhalation with the mental recitation of 'one.'

How long? Try three minutes the first time. If this is easy, then increase to five to seven minutes at each sitting. Do not set a timer. When you think the time has elapsed, glance quickly at a clock. Before long you will naturally 'internalize' the time.

To end: With eyes closed, bring your attention back to your body. Begin to wiggle your toes and fingers gently and then *very slowly* open your eyes, a little at a time. Sit for a moment or two before getting up from the chair.

This then is a simple meditation technique that carries no 'baggage' with it. You do not have to believe in any religious or spiritual precepts. No one is telling you how you should feel while doing this or what you should be thinking. Observe what is happening but please do not make any judgments about right/wrong or good/bad. Remember that even if the sitting is not an easy, relaxing experience for you, you are becoming more self-aware. You are learning important things about your body, your mind (thinking) and your emotions – this information is invaluable in your quest for optimal health. You are not like anyone else. Only you can discover what is best for you.

If this meditation technique does not work for you, or if you wish to experiment with more advanced techniques, please refer to the varieties of meditation described in Chapter 50. There you will find something suited to your individual needs.

6 DIAGNOSES: HAZARDOUS TO YOUR HEALTH OR LIFE SAVING?

Symptoms, then, are in reality nothing but the cry from the suffering organs.
- Jean Martin Charcot
The doctor may also learn more about the illness from the way the patient tells the story than from the story itself.
- James B. Herrick

The Difference Between Symptoms and Diagnosis

In Part II we will list alphabetically the most common complaints that bring people to the doctor's office. These are not diagnoses. These are what medical professionals refer to as the 'presenting complaint' or 'chief complaint.'

When a doctor or other health professional is practicing good medicine, she will listen carefully to your presenting complaint and then proceed to take a medical history. All doctors know that a carefully taken history will result in a diagnosis NINETY percent of the time. When the diagnosis is made, and shared with the patient, then therapeutic options can be discussed.

With a new patient, this process I have just described will take anywhere from one-half hour to one and one-half hours. The time needed is dependant on several variables: the patient's age, the complexity of the problem, the ability of the patient to give a good accounting, the skill and experience of the doctor.

With a returning patient, the process might take as little as fifteen minutes, depending on the same variables, *if the doctor has already reviewed the initial history and keeps all of it in mind when evaluating the patient.* If the doctor is familiar with the patient's history, but the complaint is new or complex, the time should be much longer.

When was the last time your doctor took that kind of time with you? That is, when was the last time he or she practiced good medicine on your behalf?

Chances are, whether you were a new or returning patient, you felt rushed, not heard and often misunderstood. You were probably sent for a number of laboratory tests and/or other procedures in an attempt to make a diagnosis that could have been made by you and the doctor together, alone, in the office.

If you currently have a physician or other health care provider who follows the 'good medicine' process, stick with him or her...you have found gold. If not, see if you can find such a provider or see if your practitioner can change his habits on your behalf.

Doctors will tell you that what I am suggesting here is old-fashioned, outmoded and foolish. They will tell you that such a process puts the patient at risk, that all the testing is necessary to make sure 'we are not missing something.' These comments can be roughly translated as follows, "I don't have time to take that kind of history and in any case the insurance company will not pay me for my time if I did have it. Furthermore, if I did miss something and had not done all these tests and procedures, you could sue me for malpractice."

I understand and can almost feel sympathy for the plight of most physicians practicing in 21st century America. They are not their own bosses. Their practices have become businesses, with the same bottom line as any other business, and they live in fear of being sued. Most doctors under fifty years of age have never known anything different. Well, that is really too bad, because they are missing out on the joy and satisfaction that comes when the doctor-patient relationship is one of trust and caring. This is just a guess on my part, but I believe that trusting your doctor and feeling understood and cared for will cure more ills than the prescription pad and the knife.

When is a Diagnosis Important?

Let us return now to the difference between the presenting complaint and the diagnosis. In the days when visits to the doctor were mostly about infectious disease or trauma or surgical emergencies, it was essential that the correct diagnosis be made and the patient treated appropriately. And in those situations, it is still essential today.

In these sometimes life-threatening situations, failure to make the correct diagnosis could be fatal. An experienced clinician can still make the diagnosis by history and physical alone 90% of the time. But not all doctors are that perceptive and here is where modern technological advances are often life-saving. The tests and procedures confirm the doctor's impression, or they point in another direction.

As mentioned previously, approximately 20% of all conditions require medical intervention. In these cases the doctor's knowledge and experience trumps whatever the patient may be thinking and feeling about his situation. Here is where 'putting yourself in the doctor's hands' has validity. What are these conditions? The list is extensive, but it is safe to say that almost all the problems are acute, overwhelming and life-threatening, or will become that way if intervention is not sought.

Doctors and other medical professionals need to think in terms of *diagnoses* when confronted with such patients. Patients need to know what *symptoms* or presenting complaints require medical attention as soon as possible. In our alphabetical list of complaints, we will make clear when it is essential to call the doctor. We will err on the side of caution: symptoms which *may* lead to a diagnosis of life-threatening illness will be emphasized and the course of action indicated.

Warning: Diagnoses can be hazardous to your health!

No, I am not talking here about mis-diagnosis. Diagnoses, even 'correct' ones, can be dangerous when they are for the convenience of the doctor or the insurance industry and do not adequately reflect what is really going on with the patient. This is the 80% we have referred to previously, the diseases and conditions that are either self-limited or are related to life-style, the conditions where you can do more for your health than your doctor can. Putting a label on a patient in those circumstances is dangerous for the following reasons.

First, it inhibits further thinking, insights, and evaluation of the patient's problem. Everyone thinks they now know what is wrong – the patient, the doctor, other health professionals who may see the patient, family and friends – and they assume, wrongly, that the patient just needs to follow the doctor's advice to get better.

Second, the diagnosis may instill fear in the patient. "Oh my God, I have X." Fear, especially if chronic, leads to suppression of immune function, which in turn can lead to much more serious illness.

Third, a diagnosis leads to treatments and interventions which are usually ineffective and often dangerous: prescription medications (especially if multiple drugs are used) and sometimes unproven surgical and other invasive technical procedures.

How refreshing it would be if doctors were willing to say, "You have a set of symptoms that don't fall into any useful diagnostic category. We have ruled out anything life-threatening. We need to think more about this problem. Perhaps together we can determine what is going on." Few doctors are comfortable saying this and most patients, sadly, have come to believe there is a quick fix for all their problems.

The Power of Why

A wise clinician, teacher and friend of mine once advised, 'always ask yourself why *this* patient is suffering from *this* particular condition at *this* time.'

I always like to ask the patient, why do you think you are having this problem now? I encourage them to think outside the box before trying to answer the question. Specifically, I urge them to consider reasons that don't necessarily make sense but that just feel right.

If they are under 50, I sometimes say, why does your mother think you got sick? Or, what does your spouse think is going on.

The answers I get are often revealing and lead to a useful way of looking at the problem, which is in fact a diagnosis of sorts, and can be immensely useful to the patient and me in the search for a 'cure.'

Sometimes it is relatively simple. A patient complaining of fatigue may tell me that her mother says she doesn't get enough sleep. We then explore her sleep patterns and the reasons behind her insomnia. Another patient may tell me that his wife complains that he looks angry all the time, even though he denies feeling angry. I may then explain that his chronic low back pain may well be due to repressed angry feelings and discuss what he can do about that.

At times the patient's 'hunch' about themselves, which they have been loathe to discuss with anyone else because it doesn't make sense, is right on target. A woman with severe asthma who had no known allergies and whose wheezing had been resistant to treatment told me, "I just can't help thinking that it has something to do with my son." She was talking about her only son who was sent to Iraq a few days before the onset of her asthma. This woman, by the way, experienced complete remission of her symptoms when she relaxed her 'stiff upper lip' and began to cry openly about her fears for her son.

The above examples might lead you to think that repressed or unexpressed feelings are often the cause of chronic medical problems. And you would be right. I have found that to be the case in the majority of patients with chronic disease whom I have seen over the past thirty years. But it is not always the case, and the practitioner needs to be alert to other possibilities. He or she needs to be a good detective.

One patient complained that he had to get up four or five time per night to urinate and that it was interfering with getting a good night's sleep. I thought, a-ha, a prostate problem, which any good doctor would think of first. But his prostate had already been evaluated by a urologist and found to be normal. Besides, he did not have the problem every night. I asked him to keep a written record of the items he ate and drank each evening and to correlate that with his symptoms. We discovered that on the nights he was symptomatic, he drank a cup of peppermint tea before bed, to aid digestion. Peppermint is known to be irritating to the bladder in many people. His problem resolved when he discontinued that habit.

Understanding the difference between symptoms and diagnosis is important. Then you can learn to become your own diagnostician, your own 'good doctor,' by really listening to what your body and mind and spirit are telling you. Your body is sending you messages all the time; do not ignore these 'symptoms.' During moments of quiet, take notice of the thoughts and feelings that have possessed you. Use all this information in your quest to become healthy and stay that way.

In Part II of the book, you will learn self cure methods for many common illnesses and conditions and you will learn when it is necessary to consult a licensed physician for these problems. You may have a condition that is not covered in the book; but even so, you can apply the self-awareness skills you have practiced to determine the correct path for yourself.

Part II

SELF CURE OF SPECIFIC PROBLEMS

How to use this section:

Part II includes a number of conditions, listed alphabetically, which are possible to prevent, ameliorate or cure through your own initiative. Each of the listed conditions is followed by a brief description, which is important to read so that you and I can be sure we are talking about the same thing. If the description matches your experience, you should then read on to find out the best approach to the problem. Situations in which it is important for you to consult your doctor are *italicized*.

The 'treatment' of each condition will usually be divided into three sections corresponding to our Three Pillars of health promotion and disease prevention from Part I: Intake (or Nutrition), Exercise, and Going to the Source. Please remember that, with some obvious exceptions, this is not an either/or process. It would not be wise to tell yourself, 'I'm just going to try the nutritional advice and skip the rest.' This would be defeating the whole purpose of this book, which is about an *integrated* approach to your health.

In some instances you will be told to try an exercise in another chapter. It will be easy to find and you will be given enough detail to make it effective for you.

7 ALLERGIES

Some men also have strange antipathies in
their natures against that sort of food which
others love and thrive upon. I have heard of
one that could not endure to eat either bread
or flesh; of another that fell into a swooning fit
at the smell of a rose.
- Increase Mather

Traditionally, allergies are classified according to the bodily system that is affected: respiratory, as with hay fever (runny nose, itchy eyes) and asthma; gastrointestinal reactions which are called food allergies; and skin, such as hives and contact dermatitis.

The conventional approach has been for the doctor, who is usually an allergist or a dermatologist, to do skin testing to determine what substances you are allergic to, and then prepare a vaccine to desensitize you to the effects of that allergen. Of course you also are strongly advised to avoid contact with that particular substance. This has been effective to a limited degree. However, often patients would complain that after the treatment they have then developed allergies to a number of new items that previously tested negative.

Recent research and experience indicates that most, if not all, allergic reactions begin with the gastrointestinal tract and that probably we are set-up for these allergies early in life by being fed foods that overwhelm the protective barrier of the infant's intestinal lining. It is well-known that the longer a baby is exclusively breast-fed, the less likely he is to develop allergies – not just food allergies, but respiratory and skin reactions as well.

As with almost all of the conditions we will be looking at, the old adage that an ounce of prevention is worth a pound of cure holds true here. You can't do anything about what you were fed as an infant, but you can spare your child the same problem. An infant should be breast fed for at least 3-6 months before any other foods are introduced and even then they should be introduced one at a time, slowly.

Note: Asthma has become a huge problem in our society and it is clear that most of it has little to do with the traditional concept of allergy. Therefore it merits its own category and will be found in Chapter 11.

Allergic Rhinitis (Hay Fever)

In persons with a family history or genetic predisposition, allergic rhinitis typically results from exposure to airborne allergens (irritants) such as dust mites, animal dander, mold spores and seasonal allergens such as pollen from trees, grasses, and weeds. The most common sense approach to self-care for allergies is to avoid these triggers. Here are some other things that you can do for your self that will make your life at home or outdoors easier and more comfortable during your allergy season.

Nutritional:

Following the 7 Guidelines for Eating Well in Chapter 3 helps balance the immune system's response to contact with allergens and will reduce the severity of allergic rhinitis. In addition to drinking plenty of water between meals, certain foods can be very helpful.

About 3 months before allergy season, add yogurt (preferably organic) to your diet containing a probiotic called lactobacillus acidophilus, which helps reduce allergic reactions to pollen. Buy the plain variety and add a teaspoon of locally produced honey (available at your local farmer's market or apiary). If dairy is a problem, you can also get this probiotic in other fermented products such as sauerkraut or kimchi. Raw local honey by itself or in tea is also a strong preventative and remedy for pollen allergies. Local honey contains tiny amounts of pollen (not enough to cause an allergic reaction) from the same varieties of flowering plants and grasses releasing pollen into the air you breathe. As your body becomes accustomed to these pollens, it stops over-reacting when you breathe them. Continue with a teaspoon a day through your allergy season.

Eating fresh vegetables and foods rich in Vitamins C and A is helpful year-round as is eating onions, spicy foods, dark chocolate and dishes prepared with parsley, (not sage), rosemary, and thyme, fennel, and ginger. Teas such as green, chamomile, and peppermint can be soothing and all are enhanced by local honey. All of these can help your body reduce the formation of histamine – the chemical that causes the sneezing, itchy eyes, runny nose and other allergy symptoms.

Allergies and inflammation can exacerbate each other, so eating the anti-inflammatory diet described in Chapter 52 can also help.

Remember to follow the 7 Guidelines for Eating Well in Chapter 3, and…

Avoid eating:

- Wine or grape juice, dried fruits and beer containing sulfites as these can set off an allergic attack.

Eat more:

- Local honey, especially raw and unfiltered.
- Yogurt cultured with lactobacillus acidophilus.
- Onions, garlic, green tea, red wine (organic to avoid sulfites) and dark chocolate (70%+ cocoa solids).
- Green leafy vegetables, cabbage, cauliflower, broccoli, green peppers, citrus fruits, berries, kiwi.
- Foods rich in omega-3 fatty acids, especially flaxseeds and cold water fish such as salmon and mackerel.
- Whole foods rich in Vitamins A, C, E and minerals zinc and selenium. These are antioxidants that can help your immune system function properly and reduce allergic symptoms.

Exercise:

Held emotions can make allergies worse. Try the exercises in Chapter 47 and make note for future reference any exercises that seem to reduce your allergy symptoms.

Going to the Source:

Here is a mind/body approach to desensitize yourself to the effects of these seasonal allergies. Sit in a chair in the meditation posture described in Chapter 5, close your eyes and breathe out fully three times. Visualize cool, clear water flowing gently through your nasal passages and throat, washing away all impurities and inflammation. Keep this up for one minute. Then imagine golden rays of sunshine healing the membranes of all affected areas, again for one minute. End by taking a deep breath and letting it out very slowly, through your nose if possible.

If you are an experienced meditator, try this: Meditate for at least five minutes, or until you feel you are in a deeply relaxed, peaceful state. Have an assistant approach you with a sample of the offending allergen (for example, ragweed) and bring it within a few inches of your face. Maintain your deeply relaxed state and simply be aware of your body's reaction to the substance. Have no expectations. Be a curious observer, a good scientist. Your response to this experiment will inform you what to do next.

Hives and other Allergic Skin Reactions

Skin rashes are very difficult to self-diagnose, even with all the information available on the web. Here is where a visit to an experienced dermatologist can be helpful. Most of the time they can make an accurate diagnosis quickly. Try to find one who has been in practice at least 15 years. Unfortunately, dermatologists do not have much to offer in the way of treatment – you will usually leave with a prescription for an expensive topical steroid.

If you are told that you are suffering from an acute or chronic allergic reaction of the skin, such as hives (acute) or eczema (chronic), it is probably due to a food allergy. You can use the 'observe and record' process from Chapter 3 to discover the offending agent and then eliminate it from your diet. Other nutritional approaches are outlined below.

If your acute allergic rash is accompanied by other severe symptoms such as difficulty breathing or faintness, seek medical help immediately. You could be suffering from 'anaphylactic shock' – the kind of reaction that occurs in some people after a bee sting or ingestion of peanuts.

It is useful to remember that a significant number of skin problems, especially chronic ones, are related to other underlying diseases, including mental/emotional states. This is another reason to get an accurate diagnosis from a skilled dermatologist and then, of course, to seek treatment, or administer self-care, for the underlying condition.

Gastrointestinal/Food Allergies

How are you going to know if your chronic or recurrent 'upset stomach' is due to a food allergy or to one of the other many conditions that affect the gastrointestinal tract? There is no easy answer to this and it is very unlikely that you will get much help from your doctor in this regard. Again, the best bet is to 'observe and record.' The most likely offending food substances are wheat, fish, nuts, eggs, milk and soy but it could be almost anything.

The abdominal symptoms of a food allergy are not significantly different from those of other gastrointestinal conditions. In the chapter on gastrointestinal disorders (Chapter 23) we will discuss these symptoms and how to go about making a diagnosis and instituting treatment.

If you are lucky enough to be able to identify the allergenic food substance, then the treatment is obvious: eliminate it from your diet.

8 ANGINA

My life is in the hands of any rascal who
chooses to annoy and tease me.
- John Hunter

Angina deserves a special category separate from Heart Disease, because in a significant number of people with angina, or chest pain, no heart disease can be found.

If you have severe chest pain on exertion (going upstairs, for example), see your doctor at once. Do not try any of the approaches mentioned here until your doctor tells you that you do not have heart disease.

Sometimes it is not easy to tell the difference between chest pain due to compromised circulation in the blood vessels feeding the heart and chest pain from other causes. To further complicate the issue, sometimes those vessels are clear and open but go into spasm, which feels the same and can precipitate a heart attack. The cause of this condition (called coronary artery spasm) is often unclear, but research shows that it can be brought on by an overwhelming emotion that is unexpressed, that is being squelched out of fear of behaving inappropriately.

For example, my patient Larry, a forty-seven year old construction supervisor, came to see me because of chronic pain and pressure in his chest. He was worried about a heart attack and had been referred to a cardiologist by his family doctor. The specialist told Larry that his heart was 'sound as a dollar.' His discomfort had been present for nearly three months. As we talked, Larry revealed that he and his wife had been separated by mutual agreement for the past six months. However, a few days before his chest pain began, Larry had been out walking in the evening and had come across a couple in a parked car, locked in a passionate embrace. It was his wife, with another man who was a friend of his. He had gone home and tried to put the image out of his mind, telling himself there was no reason to be upset. I worked with Larry over the next several visits to help him access his authentic feelings of rage and grief over this betrayal. I also taught him an expressive voice exercise to give voice to the heartbreak he was going through. His chest symptoms quickly subsided.

It will be worthwhile to take a closer look at the concept of heartbreak. Let us assume that you have been told by your doctor that you do not have heart disease but you continue to have chest pain in the area of your heart. Perhaps the breath and voice exercise I suggested gives you some relief, but the pain keeps recurring, or perhaps it is with you most of the day. You may be suffering from heartbreak, even if you are unaware of feeling sad, or lonely.

Heartbreak can occur in many circumstances besides the loss of a loved one. When your girlfriend breaks up with you or when your dog dies, chances are you know you are heartbroken. You *feel* bereft, sad, lonely. Tears come easily. This condition, though painful, is a perfectly normal reaction to loss and, as long as you allow the feelings to flow, will not lead to depression or physical illness such as heart disease.

We sometimes use the expression, 'I've got my heart set on…..' meaning that it is something we want very badly. I am not talking here about the acquisition of things, such as a new car or a triple chocolate dessert, but rather the desire for something that gives meaning to our lives, that enables us to pursue our dreams. Perhaps it is getting married, or going to graduate school, or getting a particular job. Or even getting a book published.

Anything that we have had our heart set on can lead to heartbreak if it does not materialize. You are left at the altar. Or you may marry that special person only to find out a few years later that it was a big mistake but now you have two kids and a lot of responsibility. You have gotten what you wanted and now you have lost it. Because these types of situations often take a long time to develop, we do not feel the pain of loss. We get on with our lives and 'forget' about what was troubling us. But our heart knows what has been lost and it may be trying to tell us something. If we constrict the muscles of our chest (unconsciously) in order to silence the messenger we may unintentionally create a dangerous situation for our health.

Constriction and tension, when chronic, can lead to a 'shut-down' of energetic flow to that area of the body, and when that happens, disease can ensue. We are focused now on heart disease, but other serious conditions can develop as well.

So when you have unexplained chest pain that your doctor says is not due to heart disease, pause for a moment. Consider that instead of running from one specialist to another, undergoing unpleasant and expensive tests and procedures, that you may be able to do more for your health than your doctor can. Sit in a chair with your eyes closed, place both hands over your heart, breathe out fully several times and wait for a message from your heart. It may come in the form of an image. Or words may pop into your head, or there may be a physical sensation. Just sit and observe what is happening. Keep your mind open to the possibilities, even if they don't make 'sense.'

If you find or even suspect that a current or past situation of loss is affecting you, try to bring it fully into your consciousness. Write about it, talk to a friend or therapist about it. See if some feelings (sadness, grief, loneliness, bitterness, rage) arise and then let those feelings flow. Just this simple process can open up channels of energy that have long been blocked and thus the reversal of the disease process begins.

I frequently hear patients say, "what is the use of re-hashing that old stuff…I can't do anything about it now…I can't really change my ….." It is very important at this point to realize that you don't have to change anything about your situation in order to regain your health. You simply have to fully feel and appropriately express the authentic emotions connected with that situation. You might not be happy, but you do not need to be sick. Then sometime in the future you may be able to change the situation.

Nutritional:

If your angina is due to partially blocked coronary arteries (as diagnosed by your physician with appropriate tests), a nutritional plus mind/body approach can be just as effective for reversing your heart disease as surgical procedures. See Chapter 25 - Heart Disease for the specific nutritional interventions. If your angina or chest pain is *not* due to blocked arteries, nutritional interventions are not likely to be helpful.

Exercise:

Everyone knows that the right kind of safe physical exercise can be helpful in reversing heart disease. What is less known is that there are many other types of exercise that can be helpful as well. Again you will find recommendations in Chapter 25 – Heart Disease.

However, here is an exercise you can safely try when you have chest pain, *provided that your doctor has told you that you do not have heart disease.* While you are having the pain, lie flat on a carpeted floor with a small pillow under your neck so that your head is slightly tilted back. Open your mouth wide, take a medium deep breath and hold it for two seconds. Then release the breath by making a loud, long sound – AHHHHHH – try to hold the sound until the very end, forcing all the air out of your lungs. Then let the breath flow back in naturally. Rest for about fifteen seconds then repeat the exercise, three times. The pain should be gone. A more advanced form of this exercise is to have another person kneel beside you and gently press down on your sternum (breast bone) all the while you are vocalizing, then release the pressure for the in-breath.

An alternative to this is the following. When you are experiencing the chest pain, force yourself to cough, hard and long, forcing all the air out of your lungs. Keep coughing until the pain subsides.

Going to the Source:

Going to the source is not appropriate during an acute episode of chest pain. But practicing the techniques under Going to the Source in Chapter 25 – Heart Disease, along with correct nutrition and exercise, can save your life.

9 ANXIETY AND PANIC ATTACKS

> *A continual anxiety for life vitiates all the
> relishes of it, and casts a gloom over the whole
> face of nature; as it is impossible we should
> take delight in anything that we are every
> moment afraid of losing.*
> - Joseph Addison

I don't know of any disease or condition that is
more misunderstood than anxiety. Doctors, patients,
and even many therapists do not understand. Everyone
thinks they know what the other person means when he
or she says they are anxious. So much so that they
rarely take time to ask the simple question: tell me what
your anxiety is like. I often phrase the question this way
– if you didn't know the word 'anxiety,' how would you
describe what you are feeling.

In answering that question, the process of healing
begins. Because the responses to the question invariably
involve a variety of somatic (body) experiences –
anything from cold feet to burning ears. I don't think
there is a physical sensation that I have NOT heard

from people when describing their anxiety. Except one: pain.

Pain is a danger signal, often indicating that something has gone wrong with the body and that an actual disease process might be present. But as patients describe all these other somatic sensations that can occur with anxiety, they begin to realize that they are not suffering from any potentially dangerous illness. Rather, they are going through something horribly unpleasant (when the anxiety is severe) and that they want relief.

Most people seek relief through medication. Whether it is self-medication through alcohol and other easily abused substances, or doctor-prescribed drugs, this route often leads to additional health problems. However, if the anxiety is mild and intermittent, a small dose of 'old-fashioned tranquilizers' is often helpful and helps to get the person through a tough time. Let's say, for example, that you have to give weekly presentations as part of your work and that this makes you nervous and that popping a valium calms your sweaty palms, racing heart and breathlessness. Fine, go for it. In this case you are using a prescribed drug on an as-needed basis and there is little danger in doing so. Chances are slim that you will become addicted, and the side-effects should be minimal when the drug is used occasionally.

If, on the other hand, you have to give *daily* presentations and it does not get easier with practice, I urge you not to use drugs but to seek out other ways to 'control' your apprehension. Find a good therapist and/or pick and choose from the variety of techniques described below.

I do not believe that panic attacks are a separate entity from severe anxiety. I think they are another manifestation of the same process leading to severe and overwhelming anxiety.

Whether you suffer from chronic anxiety, even if mild, or moderate to severe anxiety frequently, I want to caution you against taking medication on a prolonged, regular basis. There is no specific drug cure for anxiety. Penicillin cures strep throat. That is specific, you can count on it. Penicillin kills the strep bacteria and does not hurt us (unless of course you have an allergy to that drug). You will not become addicted to penicillin nor will you need larger and larger doses each time you get strep. There is no such specificity when it comes to medications used to treat anxiety and, for that matter, most of the ills that beset us in 21st century America. You will likely need larger and larger doses, develop unpleasant and sometimes dangerous side-effects, and there is a strong possibility of physical and/or psychological addiction.

As I mentioned, there is no end to the kinds of symptoms that anxiety produces. When the symptoms are severe, even the most stalwart among us are convinced we have some dread disease. And even getting reassurance from the doctor that it is 'just anxiety' and that we are not going to die from it gives us no relief. At times we almost wish we had a fatal illness to deliver us from this nightmare.

Even with severe anxiety most of us continue to do our work and meet our responsibilities, but we suffer through it. One might think, "If I had the flu, I could stay home and people would understand, but this is 'just anxiety.'" We can't even complain about it because it is so humiliating. There is no joy in our lives and rarely even a sense of satisfaction.

Before we wallow further in the mire of chronic and severe anxiety I want to call your attention to a little known fact which may startle you: *anxiety is not an emotion. It is the body's attempt to protect us from our feelings. You cannot experience a strong emotion and be anxious at the same time.*

Why do I say that anxiety is not an emotion? When we are experiencing any strong emotion, such as anger, sadness, joy, love, there is movement. Energy is flowing. And when we tell someone we feel sad, they know what we mean. Anxiety, despite the awful somatic sensations, is a shut down state. In this way, anxiety is similar to the emotion of fear. We say we are frozen with fear. But fear, in its pure state, leads to action: flight or fight. When we are afraid of something which we have no reason to fear (elevators, for example) we do not run from it or do battle with it. We endure our frozen state and then develop symptoms of anxiety as a result of not taking action, or, as a result of not allowing a more authentic emotion to surface, such as anger.

Why would the body want to protect us from our authentic feelings? Perhaps we learned a long time ago, as children, that certain of our emotions were unacceptable to our caregivers, the people we depended on for our very existence. Don't cry, big boys don't cry. Worse yet: oh, no honey, you're not angry. Or even, don't get so excited. So we learned to cut off those feelings by constricting our breath and clamping down on our muscles. This becomes habitual, part of the way we operate in the world. Those feelings are no longer available to us in our conscious state. Yet they are still there. Someone hurts us. We don't get angry. We don't even know we are angry. Instead, we become anxious as we clamp down even harder, restrict our breathing even more.

Incidentally, most people (including doctors) have the notion that when we are anxious we hyperventilate, that is, breathe too much. This is wrong. It is very rare to hyperventilate when anxious. Nearly every patient I have seen with anxiety has chronic restricted breathing, which gets worse when the level of anxiety is raised.

I have said that one can not experience a strong emotion and be anxious at the same time. Those of you who suffer from chronic anxiety can probably recall a scenario similar to this: You are going about your usual daily activities at work or home, feeling anxious, pre-occupied with those awful symptoms, hoping for relief. The telephone rings. It is someone calling to tell us that our child has been in an accident, or our mother has been rushed to the hospital. As we hurry off to be with our loved one, when we are in 'emergency' mode, the symptoms are gone, at least for the time being. If we had the presence of mind to notice our breathing at that point, we would see that we are breathing fully, probably rapidly, as we prepare to handle the situation. Our energy is mobilized. We are no longer shut down, no longer frozen.

Some of you may have had the experience of falling in love (or lust) at a time in your life when you have been very anxious. For a time at least the overwhelming desire we feel for that other person totally displaces our symptoms of anxiety. Sadly, it doesn't last as the 'honeymoon' wears off.

When we can re-discover and re-experience our authentic emotions and let them flow through us, we will no longer be anxious. You will find below, under

Exercise, several suggestions to facilitate this happening.

Nutritional:

To alleviate anxiety, it is important to begin by following the 7 Guidelines for Eating Well in Chapter 3. Be aware that episodes of increased anxiety can be caused by:

- Withdrawal from habitual use of alcohol, tobacco, caffeine, certain medications and other addictive substances including narcotics.
- Food allergies.
- The body reacting to artificial sweeteners, "flavor enhancers" and other additives in fast, junk or highly processed food.

You should make note of foods and drinks that contribute to anxiety symptoms as people's reactions vary. If refined sugar and artificial sweeteners make your anxiety worse, try to eat whole foods that do not spike blood sugar levels and avoid sweets, sweet drinks and fruit juices. Coffee, black tea, some sodas and energy drinks contain caffeine which can provoke anxiety, nervousness and insomnia and deplete the body of vitamins and minerals that help balance mood. Food allergies can also cause emotional problems if you are allergic to dairy, gluten, nightshade vegetables, nuts, eggs, grains or other foods.

It's important to eat meals slowly and consciously, paying attention to the food and enjoying the process of eating with a sense of gratitude. Shoving in fuel on the run, overeating, and drinking too much fluid with a meal can all exacerbate anxiety, as well as leading to indigestion, bloating, cramping and a decrease in the absorption of essential nutrients.

Smoking cigarettes, chewing tobacco, wearing a nicotine patch or chewing nicotine gum increases anxiety, makes the heart work harder and depletes the body of nutrients. Over the counter and prescription decongestants, anti-histamines and other drugs that contain caffeine, amphetamines, ephedra can also exacerbate mood and sleep issues. Chemical additives used in commercial food processing, preservatives and pesticides can have serious and unpredictable effects on your body. Try to eat whole unprocessed foods and organically grown fruits and vegetables are much as possible.

Remember to follow the 7 Guidelines for Eating Well in Chapter 3, and...

Avoid eating:
- Refined carbohydrates, sugar (in any form), especially high-fructose corn syrup.
- Sugar substitutes (e.g. NutraSweet, Equal, Splenda or saccharine).
- Drinks containing caffeine or alcohol and stimulant drugs.
- Preservatives and other food additives in processed foods, which can raise anxiety. Excess salt raises blood pressure and can lead to a potassium deficiency which can unbalance the nervous system.
- Monosodium Glutamate (MSG), a "flavor enhancer" found in Chinese take-out, "seasoned salt", and many processed foods. MSG can contribute to anxiety, migraines, insomnia, chest pains and other issues in some people.
- Meat from animals that have been fed or injected with hormones to accelerate growth.

This includes all grocery store meat unless it is specifically marked hormone-free. Avoid "corn-fed", "grain-fed", or "corn-finished" meat.

Eat more:

- Green tea contains essential nutrients that can calm the nerves and help with sleep and other nervous conditions. Chamomile and lemon balm teas are calming.
- Drinking unflavored sparkling water or club soda can reduce anxiety, relax muscles, and easing circulation by dilating blood capillaries.
- To balance and calm your mood, eat more foods which contribute essential nutrients such as omega 3 fatty acids, magnesium, B-vitamins, calcium, potassium, zinc, selenium and certain amino acids. Examples of these foods are asparagus, avocado, broccoli, carrots, garlic, onions, spinach and other green leafy vegetables, bananas, wild fish, oysters, eggs, molasses, walnuts, pastured beef, turkey or chicken, brown rice and lentils.
- Comfort foods that have specific calming emotional associations for you can be helpful during periods of anxiety but be careful to eat them in moderation or as a treat.

Exercise:

Vigorous exercise is always somewhat helpful in relieving the anxious state. It forces us to open our breathing, which in itself is useful. Plus, the vigorous movement of our body helps to get us unfrozen. Alas, the relief is temporary. It is not a cure. I would however, urge all of you with anxiety symptoms to pick a regular exercise program and stick to it. It may save you from the long-term ill effects that anxiety causes to our bodies.

Breathing exercises: do breath exercise number 1 in Chapter 45 every day. Please note that you may temporarily notice an increase in symptoms the first few times you do the exercise. This is a good sign. Push through it and you will find that is no longer a problem and that the exercise results in a feeling of well-being for several hours.

Expressive exercises: Do anything that 'gets your yah-yah's out.' In the privacy of your own room or car, yell, scream, shout, sing, pound, kick, dance wildly and laugh like a mad-man. Whatever you choose, keep it up for at least five minutes. Ten is better.

Expressive exercise with a partner: This one is great. Face your partner, standing about three feet apart. Stand tall, with hands on hips and assume (fake if necessary) an aggressive posture. You say YES, your partner responds NO, getting faster and louder each time. Using only your voice, try to convince the other to back down. Keep it up at least three minutes. Notice the remarkable relief of your symptoms.

Going to the Source:

I have explained earlier that meditation is an antidote to the effects of stress. It can also provide almost magical relief from the symptoms of anxiety while you are doing it. Use the techniques described in Chapter 5 to get yourself into a meditative state (or as one of my mentors describes it, to elicit the relaxation response). Usually you will experience nearly complete alleviation of your symptoms. Use the technique for short periods (7-10 minutes) several times a day to get relief. You will also be doing good things for your overall health and well-being in the process.

For the few of you who experience a worsening of symptoms when you sit down to meditate, don't despair. Here is an approach that will help you. First, do the breath exercise mentioned above and follow that with at least one expressive exercise. Then sit down to meditate. When you notice that the symptoms flare up at this point, turn your attention to your breath. Exaggerate the out-breath, the exhalation. Make it last as long as you can and try to make some sound along with the out-breath. A good one is the sound of Om that is often chanted in yoga classes. Hold the sound as long as the breath lasts, pause for a moment, then begin again. Let your symptoms dance and yell in your head and/or body while you continue to give all your attention to the out-breath. Keep this pattern up for at least five minutes to get relief.

While you are in the meditative state, take the opportunity to learn something about why you are anxious. I do not mean analyze the problem as if you were a therapist. Your focus here should be on what authentic emotion you might be feeling that your body is fighting against by producing the anxious state. For example, try to visualize yourself angry, perhaps in a rage at someone. What do you 'see?' Or perhaps you might be feeling despair and see yourself crying and sobbing in the arms of someone you can trust. Make these images as real as possible and notice what effect that has on your bodily symptoms.

While you are in the process of trying these techniques to help yourself, it is very important to abandon yourself to irrationality. Forget any notion you might have that things have to 'make sense' or that you have to be reasonable. Think of yourself as a little bit nuts or, if this helps, as a teenager[4].

If you get relief of your symptoms from meditation, please do yourself a favor and make it a life-long process. Do not use it "as needed". Be a committed practitioner and reap the benefits forever.

This is a book about Self Cure, but it is important here to say a few words about the role of psychotherapy in the treatment of anxiety. All 'shrinks' can help with mild or intermittent anxiety, but few know how to help those folks with severe chronic anxiety.

If the self cure methods are not helping you, you have two choices at this point. You can go the 'drug route' by finding a reputable 'psychopharmacologist' (the fancy word now used for psychiatrists whose practices are limited to prescribing medications) and taking the meds that he or she prescribes. I recommend this as a last resort only.

The other choice is to make a careful search for a therapist who does 'body-oriented psychotherapy.' This person could be an MD (psychiatrist), a PhD (psychologist) or someone with a masters degree in psychotherapy. Do NOT choose someone on the basis of their degree. Make your choice based on their training, experience and reputation. And do not hesitate to ask for an initial trial session (for which of course you will have to pay) to see if you and this person

---

[4] A note here about teenagers who are clinically anxious: I have seen and treated many of these suffering kids and I can say, without exception, that they have all been 'good kids' who are way too grown up for their chronological age. In other words, even at this early age, they have already stuffed their authentic feelings to the point that they deny their very existence.

'click.' *An experienced body-oriented psychotherapist will understand your symptoms and be able to help you with them.*

Anxiety in pre-teenaged children:

If your young child suffers from what you believe is anxiety and/or panic attacks, it is essential to intervene right away in order to prevent a life-long pattern from developing.

In the case of a very young child (less than five or six, although I have seen it work with children as old as ten), you can probably do more for him than any doctor or therapist can, provided that you can find a calm, centered place within yourself while assisting the child. *Do not attempt to help the child if you are feeling anxious.* If your spouse or one of the grandparents has a very close relationship with your anxious child and can remain calm, teach the following method to him/her.

Sit upright in a soft, comfortable chair or sofa with enough pillows behind your back and neck to prevent slouching. Place the child in your lap, facing away from you, and enfold him in your arms, gently pulling him against your chest. Say very little, but something like 'you and mommy are going to sit together for awhile and relax.' Then, take a few long slow breaths and relax your entire body as much as possible. Begin to hum softly and sing a baby's lullaby, if you know one. Maintain the relaxed state and the humming or singing for about ten minutes or until the child struggles to get free. Repeat this procedure two or three times a day.

If your child is older or repeatedly struggles against the relaxation exercise, here is another approach. Take the child for a walk in the woods, where there are no distractions other than the sights and sounds of nature. Avoid engaging him in conversation, saying, 'mommy

likes to be quiet when she is walking in the woods.'
Walk for about a half hour and if this has a calming
effect on your child, do it at least three times a week. If
he becomes anxious when returning home, encourage
him to spend a few minutes several times a day
picturing himself in the woods with you.

*If neither of these methods is successful, I would encourage
you to seek help from a body-centered psychotherapist.*

10 ARTHRITIS AND ARTHROPATHIES (JOINT DISEASE)

*Screw up the vise as tightly as possible – you
have rheumatism; give it another turn, and
that is gout.*
Anonymous

The vast majority of people suffering from arthritis
can significantly improve their condition through self-
care. *Some conditions however are best treated by going to your
doctor. The latter include: congenital and genetic varieties of joint
disease, arthritis due to acute trauma (usually a sports injury),
some forms of arthritis due to repetitive trauma, septic arthritis
(due to infection), the acute form of gouty arthritis or any acute
process where the joint is swollen, red and hot.*

But the vast majority of problems that affect the
joints do respond to self-care and prevention. These fall
into the two categories of osteoarthritis (also called
degenerative arthritis) and rheumatoid arthritis. The
former has been thought to be due to 'wear and tear' on
the joints while rheumatoid is classified as an 'auto-
immune disorder.' Neither of these explanations has

ever made sense to me. Osteoarthritis is frequently seen in people who have done little or no exercising throughout their lives. If the wear and tear theory were true, they should be free of joint problems. And the term 'auto-immune' means that our own bodies are mounting an attack against parts of ourselves. That label does not provide an explanation for this bizarre occurrence.

We get a clue as to the origin of these two disease processes if we consider that arthritis occurs with a prevalence of 15% (some authorities say 20%) of people in this country. Any condition that affects one in every five or six people, to my way of thinking, has to be a consequence of how we live our lives. Call it a life-style disease or a disease of civilization. I have seen the same percentage figures quoted for anxiety, depression and hypertension, which are more clearly related to life-style.

Let's re-state what we mean by the term life-style. Basically, it is how we live our lives. Some of it is not our choice, or at least not our individual choice, such as polluted air and water. There are other determining factors about which we do have a choice. For example, no one is forcing us to eat an unhealthy diet. We do have control over what kind and how much physical exercise we get. And, if we dig a little deeper, we will find that we do not have to live with so much stress at work and at home. We do have a choice about these things and yes, changing them would mean a monumental shift in our life-style. But it is very naïve, in my opinion, to believe that we can choose to live an unhealthy life-style and expect the medical profession to rescue us from the consequences of that choice. They are happy to take on that task. An entire industry has been built around doing just that and a lot of people get rich from our poor choices. But doctors are usually very intelligent and many of them are thoughtful individuals, and deep down they know that we have to rescue ourselves.

When it comes to the self-care of arthritis, it should be obvious that prevention is the key: healthy diet, moderate exercise, and stress-reduction. With a chronic condition like arthritis, treatment is much harder than prevention. But there is a lot that can be done, as outlined below.

Nutritional:

To prevent or ease arthritis, start by eating a healthy, balanced diet of whole foods, drink plenty of water and maintain a healthy weight. Excess weight puts extra stress on joints, and body fat produces hormones and chemicals that increase inflammation. Eat foods that tend to reduce inflammation. Drinking plenty of water helps flush out toxins and allows your body to make more of the fluid which lubricates the joints.

Eat foods rich in omega-3 fatty acids to decrease inflammation and suppress the production of chemicals and enzymes that erode cartilage. Sufferers of rheumatoid arthritis who increase consumption of omega-3's report greater strength and reduced fatigue, joint swelling, tenderness, stiffness and pain. Omega-3s seem to be less helpful for osteoarthritis, but they are not harmful. Follow the 7 Guidelines for Eating Well in Chapter 3 for a diet rich in omega-3's and Chapter 52 for an anti-inflammatory diet.

Vitamin C is a powerful antioxidant which helps the body control rheumatoid and infection-related inflammation. The body also needs Vitamin C to make collagen, the main protein in joint tissue and bone. Be sure to get enough Vitamin C by eating lots of C-rich fruits and vegetables. Megadose supplements of Vitamin C can make osteoarthritis symptoms worse, so avoid these if they cause you problems. Also take care with grapefruit if you are on blood pressure medication. Other powerful antioxidants which lower the risk of developing arthritis are found in abundance in red peppers, pumpkins, winter squash, persimmons, tangerines, papayas, corn, oranges, apricots, green leafy vegetables and yellow/orange fruits.

Ginger is an anti-inflammatory which eases arthritis pain in some people. Try using sliced or diced fresh organic ginger in stews, soups, pie crust, and homemade ice cream. You can also boil fresh ginger in water and use this infusion as a tea or use it to enhance other drinks. Ginger can act as a blood thinner, so take care with its use if taking a blood-thinning medication (even aspirin). Turmeric, the main ingredient in yellow curry, is another effective anti-inflammatory spice. Foods like green tea and red onions which contain a powerful antioxidant and anti-inflammatory are also helpful, as are berries and other richly colored fruits and vegetables.

Exercise:

Once you have either of the common varieties of arthritis, it becomes difficult to exercise. It is certainly unpleasant and probably harmful to do weight-bearing exercise when the ankles, knees or hips are involved. There are many types of non-weight bearing exercise, such as swimming, that can be very helpful. I would encourage you to seek the advice of a physical therapist, chiropractor or personal trainer about what type of exercise would be best for you.

Yoga: Gentle yoga, taught by an instructor who knows how to individualize the process (some call it yoga therapy), can be very helpful. It will be necessary for you to practice at home on a daily basis once you learn the postures and the procedure.

Hydrotherapy: While not strictly an exercise, this self-treatment can be very helpful, especially in osteoarthritis. Hydrotherapy is a time-honored discipline practiced by professionals, mostly in Europe. It can be adapted for use at home. Basically, it involves the application of warm/hot water to the affected area, followed by cold. Search the internet for details but a simple routine that I have found helpful is as follows: Soak the affected joint(s) in a basin of hot water for three minutes. The water should be hot enough to be initially uncomfortable but not so hot that it burns the skin. Follow this immediately with one minute of icy cold water. Repeat this process one or two more times.

Depending on the involved joint, it may be easier to do this with a shower hand spray or even by wrapping with wet towels, but the latter is difficult without professional equipment.

What you will probably notice is that there is nearly complete relief from the pain and an improvement in the mobility of the joint for a while after the hydrotherapy. This is not a cure, but if done regularly can result in improved function.

Deep Relaxation: I have noticed that chronic tension in the musculature is associated with arthritis in some cases. This is especially common in the back and neck but I have seen it with shoulder pain as well. Tension is very obvious in so-called TMJ (temporal-mandibular joint) where the jaws muscles are rigidly set.

To achieve deep relaxation of the muscles it is first necessary to become more aware of the tension. Try this experiment right now. Hold a tennis ball in your right hand; squeeze it as hard as you can for as long as you can. Then release the tension, let the ball drop and rest your hand in your lap. Now notice the feeling in that hand compared to the left. The right hand will be deeply relaxed.

Full body relaxation: Lie on a comfortable but firm mat on the floor. Put a small pillow under your head or neck, whichever feels better. Begin by tensing the muscles of your feet and, while holding that, progressively tighten the muscles of your legs, pelvis, abdomen, chest, back, hands, arms and shoulders, neck, face and scalp. Keep breathing while holding the tension for as long as you can. Then release the tension slowly, starting with your feet, and let the relaxation spread upwards into the rest of your body.

When you have released all the tension in your body, feel the 'letting go' sensation and let it get deeper and deeper each time you exhale. Close your eyes and imagine that you are sinking into the mat, letting go more and more. Try to 'see' and feel the profound relaxation of all your muscles and joints. Maintain that restful posture for at least three minutes. When you get up off the floor, try to carry that relaxed feeling with you for a few moments. If this exercise provides you with some relief of the discomfort of your arthritis, do it on a daily basis.

It has been my observation (not supported by any research that I know of) that patients with rheumatoid arthritis are frequently very unexpressive people. In these people, diligent practice of a variety of the expressive exercises in Chapter 47 can help to provide significant relief of symptoms. Remember, the free flow of energy and feeling through the body is a very healing process.

Going to the Source:

Meditation is an antidote to the effects of stress on your body. So to the extent that you believe that your life stresses are a factor in your arthritis, meditation will be helpful. Another good reason to meditate if you have rheumatoid arthritis, an auto-immune disorder, is that meditation enhances immune function. If you already have arthritis, you may find it painful or too challenging to sit on the floor or a meditation cushion. You can meditate just as well sitting on a chair. Meditation practice over the long-term should improve your arthritis symptoms. When beginning, it may take six weeks or more for you to notice these changes. But I encourage you to keep practicing.

11 ASTHMA

Some folk seem glad even to draw their breath.
- William Morris

The incidence of asthma in the population has increased markedly over what it was a generation ago. It used to be considered as one manifestation of allergies, along with hay fever and hives. It also seemed to have a strong 'psychogenic' component; that is, that psychological distress could bring on an attack. In addition, it was unusual for adults to develop asthma if they did not have childhood asthma.

Now all that seems to have changed. Many adults develop severe asthma. Many people of any age have asthma regardless of their tendency to allergies or their psychological make-up. It is logical to assume that much or most of the increase has to do with our polluted environment and there are certainly studies which bear that out.

I believe that the intake of toxins in our food plus the very poor nutritional quality of most people's diets these days is another culprit. Overall, I encourage anyone with a tendency to asthma to avoid pollution of any kind – air, water, food, animal dander – to the extent possible but I am not unrealistic about how far most of us can go with that approach.

Before we move on to specific self-care techniques for asthma, it is important to be aware that not all breathing difficulty is 'asthmatic.' Yes, we are 'short of breath' during an asthmatic attack, but there are many medical reasons for shortness of breath. Asthma refers specifically to difficulty getting the air out. The patient is struggling to get the air out through narrowed respiratory passages. The reason that an injection of epinephrine (adrenalin) provides instant relief is that one of the effects of that drug is to expand these passages, allowing air to flow more freely. In addition, the steroids so often prescribed for asthma produce a reduction in the inflammation of those passages, which also provides relief. Of course, both drugs are dangerous and cannot be used long-term.

The self-care treatment of asthma of psychogenic origin will be detailed at the end of the section on asthma.

Nutritional:

Following the 7 Guidelines for Eating Well in Chapter 3 will establish a basis for the nutritional treatment of asthma. Asthma is an inflammatory disease and there is evidence that eating more omega 3 fatty acids and an anti-inflammatory diet as described in Chapter 52 can be helpful. Cutting out fast food containing trans fats and making sure that the body gets enough saturated fats can bring significant improvement. The airspaces in the lungs are normally coated with a thin layer of lung surfactant, which is made up primarily of saturated fatty acids. Eating trans fats (partially hydrogenated oils) or too much omega 6 from grain-fed animals and unsaturated fat from cheap vegetable oils can lead to surfactant damage, and can increase both the incidence and severity of asthma attacks.

Some foods may bring on asthma attacks, while other foods can help to lessen or prevent attacks. If eating certain foods is followed by an asthma attack, then those foods need to be avoided. Keep a food journal and look for patterns. Some of the most common food-allergy asthma triggers are: eggs, nuts, milk, sulfites, soy, fish and chocolate. Other foods also can help guard against asthma attacks. Antioxidant vitamins A, C, and E (found in most fresh vegetables and fruits); lycopene (found in red fruits and vegetables like tomatoes); and selenium (found in Brazil nuts and grass fed meats) are among these.

The calcium, magnesium and enzymes found in raw milk if you have access to it (or raw milk cheeses if you don't) promote calmer lungs and better airflow. Regular pasteurized milk can actually become a trigger that worsens asthma attacks. Magnesium can also be found in leafy greens like spinach.

Many people with asthma also have GERD (reflux of stomach acid). Obesity and over-eating can worsen asthma and GERD, so try to maintain a healthy weight. Eat smaller meals and cut down on alcohol and caffeine when experiencing asthma symptoms.

Avoid eating:
- Fast foods, convenience foods, snacks high in sugar and salt, grain-fed meat or farm-raised fish and trans fats, hydrogenated oils, margarine

or vegetable shortening. There's some evidence that eating omega-6 fats and trans fats may worsen asthma.

- Sulfites in non-organic wine, beer, grape juice, dried fruits or sprayed salad bars, shrimp and lobster in seafood bars, or added to dough and food starches.
- Specific foods that trigger asthma for you. Common culprits are eggs, nuts, milk, sulfites, soy, fish and chocolate although your reaction will vary.
- Extremes (e.g. too much, too hot, too cold, too spicy) can trigger attacks.

Eat more:
- Fruits and vegetables, especially red fruits like grapes and tomatoes for lycopene, watercress and squash for vitamin A, leafy greens for magnesium, broccoli, cabbage, cauliflower, citrus fruits and berries for vitamin C, sweet potato, avocado and spinach for vitamin E.
- Better quality protein and fats including omega-3 fatty acids found in wild salmon, tuna, pastured meat and poultry, sardines, flaxseed. These are anti-inflammatory and help body maintain proper lung surfactant.
- Spices, nuts, chocolate, and tea, which are also rich sources of magnesium, can help reduce asthma symptoms, but take care to note if any of these are asthma triggers for you.

Exercise:
I am unaware of any form of vigorous physical exercise that would be helpful in either prevention of

asthma or relief from an attack. In fact, exercise, especially in cold weather, at times makes it worse. However, specific breathing techniques can help you become aware of your breathing patterns and improve your asthma symptoms.

Breath and Voice Exercises: Any of the breath and voice exercises detailed in Chapter 45 will be helpful in the *prevention* of an asthma attack if you perform them on a regular basis. Here is one which often can interrupt the onset of an attack if you feel one coming on. Try it at the first sign that your breathing is becoming difficult.

Lie on your back on a firm mattress or on the floor. Place a rolled up towel under your shoulder blades so that your head is tilted back somewhat. Take a medium deep breath, hold it for two seconds, then release it with a long, loud sound….AAAAAAH. Try to keep the voice going as long as there is any breath left in your lungs. When you reach the end, rest for a few seconds, then repeat the sound. Do this ten times.

This exercise is essentially the same as the one outlined above for relief for chest pain. At times it may not be possible to lie on the floor and of course you cannot always be in a place where you can release that much sound. One very safe place is in your car. When you are driving with your windows closed, no one can hear any sounds you make. Simply arch your back a little, take the breath as instructed and let the sound flow.

The following practice from an experienced yoga teacher can also give relief. Since asthma is often characterized by difficulty breathing out, yoga postures which accentuate the exhale can help to lessen an attack or simply ease constricted breathing. For example, try to relax in a supported forward bend, head supported by yoga blocks or pillows high enough to make the posture very comfortable. Imagine softening the diaphragm and muscles around the lungs so that the breath, even if limited, slides out on its own. Continue this practice as long as it is helpful, so long as you can remain comfortable and relaxed.

Going to the Source:

Anyone who has had the experience of not getting enough air knows that there is a tendency to panic. Breath is essential to life, so breathing difficulty feels like a life or death situation. Panic, in turn, leads to further difficulty getting air. If the situation is not dire, meditation can effectively eliminate the panic component of the problem, providing significant relief and reassurance.

Sit in a meditative posture. Try to relax your body if possible. Turn your attention to your breath. Do not try to change your breathing in any way. This is very important. Any effort on your part to 'do something' will make it worse. Simply sit and observe your breath coming in and going out. If you can remain simply observant and detached from the outcome, you will notice a significant improvement in your breathing after a few minutes.

A few words on Childhood Asthma:

When children wake up in the middle of the night with an asthmatic attack, the response of the parents can make the problem worse or better. If the parent responds with panic or anxiety in her voice or movements, the child's asthma worsens. On the other hand, calmly holding the child on one's lap while talking softly in a reassuring manner can relax the child and lessen the severity of the attack.

If the child's breathing becomes very labored and he or she is gasping for air, medical attention should be sought immediately.

During cold weather, it often helps to bundle up the child and carry her outside into the cold, moist air. Again, a calm, reassuring attitude will also help.

Self-care of asthma of psychogenic origin:

This is not intended to sound like blaming the victim. When something is described as being of psychogenic origin or having a psychogenic component it does not mean that the person is 'crazy' or has serious psychological problems. We all have our ways of being in the world. Some of us are very expressive with our emotions and others are more reserved. When it comes to the role of our feelings as contributors to our physical ailments, the expressive person is better off. As I have said before, when energy and feeling flow freely through the body, our health is enhanced. Holding back involves muscular contraction, usually chronic, and this eventually creates stagnation and disease.

The most effective way to control our feelings is to restrict our breathing. The process is of course unconscious. This can lead to a number of respiratory problems, among them a tendency to asthma.

Breathing exercises will help in this situation, but not much. The reserved person will unwittingly control the breath even while doing the exercise. On the other hand, use of the voice can be remarkably healing. There are voice exercises listed in Chapter 45 and I encourage you to try these. But even more effective is anything that comes out of your mouth with energy and spontaneity. Sing your heart out. Sing clear and loud and long. Shout and swear in the privacy of your room or car. Keep it up for ten minutes. Laugh like a madman for five minutes. And above all, if you possibly can, cry as if your heart is broken. Wail and sob until you are drained. You will then breathe freely and easily.

12 LOW BACK PAIN

Radiographs and magnetic resonance imaging (MRI) for patients with lower back pain are associated with increased cost, poorer health in recipients, and an increased risk for surgery.
- Chou R, Qaseem A, Owens DK, Shekelle P. advice for high-value health care from the American College of Physicians. Ann Intern Med. 2011;154(3):181-189.

Almost everyone in the modern, industrialized world gets a backache at one time or another. It is so common, especially in men, that everyone knows, or thinks they know, what we are talking about when we complain about our backs. Oh yeah, they say, I've had that too, it's probably your mattress. Backache has been attributed to mattresses that are too soft, or ones that are too hard; to not enough exercise, or too much exercise; to poor posture; to heavy lifting or lifting with poor posture; to prolonged standing or prolonged sitting. There is some truth in all of these assumptions, and none of it is helpful.

The sort of backache where we are able to continue with our daily activities should probably not be thought of as a medical problem at all. It certainly is not something requiring medical intervention. An occasional over-the-counter pain killer and a bit of rest and relaxation is all that's required. However, if your back pain is accompanied by sciatica (pain shooting down the leg), this indicates that a disc is bulging, dislocated or possibly even ruptured, and impinging upon the nerves running through the back. In this case, it is imperative to rest. Cut way back on daily activities even if it is possible to do them because for long-term back health, it is much better to give the body time to heal. If you normally run 10 miles a day, try walking one mile instead.

Clinical studies prove that rest and time heal the majority of back injuries equally as effectively and as quickly as any other type of intervention (e.g. surgery, chiropractic care, medication). After two weeks of rest the sciatica should resolve – assuming that you have not reinjured yourself in that time by doing too much. If not, it may be worthwhile to ask your doctor for a referral to a physical therapist for some exercises.

ON THE OTHER HAND, there is this scenario, familiar to quite a number of you: you are bending over to tie your shoe and suddenly you find yourself on the floor with excruciating pain in your lower back. Any movement intensifies the pain from a level 10 to a something off the charts. Somehow you manage to inch your way into a position on the floor that allows you to breathe and the pain is tolerable as long as you don't move any part of your body except perhaps your head and hands. You know from prior experience that without a high dose of narcotics you'll be in this position for a very long time, certainly hours and maybe a few days.

This is the variety of back pain we are addressing in this section. It should probably be called Back Spasm, for in fact that is what precipitates the pain. When you are in the acute phase of such spasm and pain, you have little choice except to medicate, orally, topically or by injection. Application of nearly continuous ice packs will help, but if you want or need to return to work, you will need a prescription of some kind. Beyond that, your doctor is of little use in this situation. I have known several people who have been helped by chiropractic intervention during this acute phase, but I have known more who have not been. It may depend upon the skill of the individual practitioner.

Once you have gotten past the acute spasm and excruciating pain and are moving cautiously about, interventions by chiropractors, acupuncturists, massage and physical therapists may be somewhat helpful. Notice that I have not included here a visit to the orthopedic surgeon. Although popular for many decades in the past (with no research data to back it up), back surgery, even for a 'slipped-disc,' is a bad idea. It is no more effective than non-surgical interventions and may cause you lasting harm.

For those of you who suffer chronic and/or recurrent episodes of back spasm, here is an important piece of information which can be very helpful: Back spasm which occurs for no apparent reason (i.e. you have not tried to lift the front end of a Volkswagen) is *always preceded by chronic underlying tension in the muscles of the low back.* If you reject this notion, do not bother to read on. If you accept it, then the good news is that the debilitating back spasm episodes can actually be prevented by resolving the underlying chronic muscular tension. The rest of this section will be devoted to helping you discover the reasons for the underlying tension *in your case* and some suggestions for relief of that tension. In this instance, we will reverse the usual order of our Three Pillars and deal first with Going to the Source.

Going to the Source:

Sit for a moment and think about someone you know who, like you, suffers from this agonizing kind of back pain. Chances are the person you have in mind is, like you, a nice guy, responsible, hard working; not a slacker, not a mean sonofabitch.

Neither he, nor you, deserves this kind of pain.

Now go deeper. Preferably use the meditation technique you learned in Chapter 5 to elicit the 'relaxation response.' Notice how it feels to be in this state. Ask yourself if you think you would be subject to acute back spasm if you could go about your daily routines while remaining in this state.

I suspect you are thinking, fine, but what's the use of it. I can't get anything done in this state. If I stayed this way I might not even want to get anything done. BINGO. You have now found the key to begin an examination of how you live your life. Nothing short of that path will be of use in preventing your back pain. Because the chronic tension (accompanied inevitably by low-grade chronic inflammation) in your low back occurs as a result of your not-knowing. It is not much about what you are *doing* on a day to day basis. It is about *not knowing how you feel* about it and not finding an outlet for those feelings.

I can hear you saying, oh, I *know* that I don't like all that responsibility, but I have to do it. So, wouldn't it be better to find a way to not feel it as a burden, perhaps even to enjoy it? Yes, it most certainly would, and if your attitudinal shift was real, and not an affirmation layered on top of deep resentment, it certainly would free up your tension and prevent further episodes of back pain and many other ailments as well. It would be the kind of personal growth everyone hopes for and few attain.

The next best option is this. Realize that *knowing is not the same as feeling.* You might 'know' you are sad because your dog died, but if you don't feel that sadness and express it, you are in for trouble. So knowing that you don't like all that responsibility is not going to help you.

The key is this. You can remain a nice, responsible guy as long as you and someone else you trust knows that you are not really such a nice guy and that you hate all that f*#**# responsibility and that you are damned angry about it. Feel all that, every day if necessary, and your chronic tension will melt away. When you are aware of and express your anger and resentment, you are not (literally) holding anything back, you are not storing those emotions in your muscles. In good time and in a responsible manner, you probably will find a way to alter your approach to work and other responsibilities so that you can live your life in a way that allows for more pleasure and less pain.

I have used responsibility to illustrate the situation, but resentment about almost anything in your life can result in the same process. Dissatisfaction in the marriage, an unfair boss, financial problems – all of these and more can result in chronic tension in your muscles if you are unaware of your real feelings and/or fail to express them.

I wish there were short-cuts to the above process, methods that you might use to get rid of, once and for all, that pain in the back. Surgery is not the answer, narcotics and other medications give short term relief but can be hazardous. Interventions by alternative practitioners such as acupuncture and chiropractic and massage provide safe but temporary amelioration of the pain and spasm and I encourage you to try these approaches, but do not expect a cure.

The most effective self-care for back spasm and pain has already been detailed above. In addition, there are a few exercises that I have found helpful. These exercises *should only be done when you are free of noticeable pain and spasm.* If you begin to feel pain during the performance of these exercises, stop at once, apply some ice, and rest.

Exercise:

The exercises detailed below are designed to assist in freeing up chronic tension in the low-back. You can try any or all of them, gently at first, and with very mindful attention to the movements of your body as you perform the exercise.

Partial leg kicks: Lie on a very firm mattress or a thick mat on the floor with a small pillow under your head. Bend your knees so that your feet are flat against the mat. Bring your right foot up in the air as far as is comfortable (i.e., you are straightening your leg), hold briefly, then drop it back down, 'slapping' the mat with the sole of your foot. Then do the left leg in the same manner. Keep this up, increasing the number of kicks and the speed of your kicking, until you are fatigued.

Then rest deeply for a couple of minutes before getting up. If you find this helpful, try to slowly increase the number of kicks each day, working up to at least 100.

Full leg kicks: Position yourself on the mat as above. Lie flat with both legs extended (i.e., knees not bent), resting on the mat. Keep your hands at your sides. Slowly 'draw' your right leg up, dragging your heel along the mat until the knee is fully bent, then lift your foot toward the ceiling as far as you can. Hold it there for a moment, then bring it down hard, a straight-leg kick into the mat, so that your heel and the entire back of your leg hits the mat at the same time. Then repeat the process with the left leg. Keep it up, alternating legs, until you are tired. Both the partial and full leg kick exercises will be greatly enhanced if you release your breath with each kick – count ONE out-loud, with some force, with the first leg, then TWO with the second, then back and forth. Slowly, over several days, see if you can work up to 50.

Stand, bend and shake: Stand in bare feet with your feet parallel and about nine inches apart. Bend your knees slightly (so they are not locked). Slightly shift your weight onto the balls of your feet, but make sure your heels stay in contact with the floor. Stand in this position for at least three minutes, letting yourself relax into it, breathing freely and easily, letting go of tension in your body, especially your jaw and belly – let the jaw and belly 'hang.'

Then gradually bend from the hips (not the waist) with your hands hanging down in front of you as if your aim was to touch your toes. Make sure your weight stays on the balls of your feet and that your head drops along with your body. Release any tension in your neck so that your head can 'flop' down. Be sure to keep the knees bent. In fact, bend them more, if necessary, so that your hands can get closer to the floor. Stay in this hanging over position for at least a minute. If you are lucky, your legs will begin to shake, or vibrate, as the tension is released. Try to increase the vibration by gently bending and straightening the knees. While doing this, keep the weight on the balls of your feet. Do not rock back on your heels.

After a minute or so, come back up to a standing position very slowly, exaggerating your breathing so that you do not get dizzy. If you have managed to start some vibrations in the legs, let that shaking continue in the standing position. Alternate back and forth between standing and bending, three times. Your goal is to get as much vibration in the legs as possible.

Pelvic bounce: When there is low back tension, the pelvis does not move freely. This exercise will help to free-up the pelvis and release tension in the back.

Lie on a firm mat on the floor with a small pillow under your head or neck. Place a small rolled up towel cross-wise in the hollow between your back and pelvis. Only an inch or two of thickness is required. Bend your knees so that your feet are flat against the mat. Press your feet into the mat just enough so that that your pelvis is slightly lifted off the mat, no more than an inch. Then release the pressure so that your pelvis (your buttocks) slaps down onto the mat. Repeat this, slowly at first, then more rapidly. The image I like to use it that of a basketball being dribbled very close to the floorboards. Like the ball, let the pelvis develop a bouncing action of its own, almost as if you are not doing it. Keep this up for two or three minutes, as long as it feels free and easy.

In addition to the mechanical exercises listed above, you will find it very helpful to practice a series of Expressive Exercises, which will help you unlock the feelings which have been 'stored' in the muscles of your low back. These exercises are detailed in Chapter 47 – Expressive Exercises. Pay special attention to the anger releasing exercises using the voice. Once you have given voice to your hidden feelings, you will find ways to safely and sanely express these feelings in social and work situations. Be patient. It will take months to effect changes in your mind/body sufficient to prevent further episodes of back pain.

Nutritional:
The nutritional interventions for this condition would be the same as those suggested for chronic inflammation. Try the Anti-inflammatory diet outlined in Chapter 52.

13 BAD BREATH

Let me repeat it: if you cannot bear to be told
by your bosom friend that you have a strong
breath, you deserve not to have a friend.
- Johann Kaspar Lavater

While not an actual disease, this condition is more troubling for those close to the patient than to the individual himself. Often, the afflicted person is unaware of the problem and needs to be told. Spouses will usually convey such information but others, even close friends, are loath to offend. If you suspect you have offensive breath, have the courage to ask someone who will be honest with you. Beyond the social implications, bad breath can be a sign of underlying pathology.

Bad breath has its origins in either the respiratory system or the gastrointestinal tract. It can come from the mouth (gingivitis, tooth decay, dentures), the stomach or small intestine when the digestive process is impaired. It can emanate from a sinus infection or a post-nasal drip or from the lower respiratory passages secondary to infection. It can also come from the lungs as in the 'acetone' breath of starvation.

In traditional Chinese medicine and in Ayurvedic medicine, practitioners are trained to make diagnoses based partially on the odor of the breath. If you have bad breath and are not getting help from conventional dentists or doctors, I encourage you to seek out an experienced alternative healer.

Nutritional:

Bad breath can be caused by bacterial or viral infections in the mouth, throat, nose, sinuses or stomach, digestive issues, residual food on the teeth and using tobacco, alcohol, coffee or other highly acidic drinks. Following the 7 Guidelines for Eating Well in Chapter 3 is the best place to start for avoiding or curing bad breath. Bad breath may also signal other conditions such as diabetes, ulcers, GERD (acid reflux), kidney, liver or respiratory disorders. Stress, dehydration and allergies can trigger episodes of bad breath.

Certain foods such as strong cheeses, canned fish, processed meats, garlic, onions and curry spices are frequently cited as cause for bad breath. Keep a food journal and note which foods cause problems for you.

Poor digestion, constipation, or bowel disorders may contribute to bad breath. Try not drinking during meals in order not to dilute your stomach acid. This should improve digestion. A tablespoon of apple cider vinegar before meals can also help. Eating green leafy vegetables and fruits containing digestive enzymes, especially kiwi, papaya and pineapple can be helpful too.

Vitamin deficiencies (especially vitamin C and niacin) and lactose intolerance can also cause bad breath. Eating more vegetables and fruits as well as probiotics (available in yogurt and fermented foods such as sauerkraut) also aids digestion and reduces acid reflux, yeast overgrowth, or intestinal fermentation which can lead to bad breath.

Immediate relief from bad breath can be had by brushing, flossing and rinsing with water. Toothpaste with baking soda or tea tree oil, and adding dilute hydrogen peroxide to your rinse eliminates bacteria and can keep breath fresh for several hours. Most commercial mouthwashes contain alcohol, which will make matters worse after the minty scent wears off. A better mouthwash is tomato juice. Other effective food remedies are chewing parsley, fresh mint, filberts (hazelnuts), alfalfa sprouts, anise, cardamom, dill, sage or fennel seeds or leaves, or drinking fenugreek, clove or mint tea. Sucking a lemon sprinkled with salt will alleviate garlic or onion breath.

In my experience, the most common form of bad breath is 'morning breath.' If you have foul breath upon awakening an instant cure is the following. Cut an apple into thin slices. Sprinkle lemon juice and a bit of grated ginger root on the slices and eat them, chewing well. This works much better than brushing your teeth or using mouthwash.

Avoid:
- If possible, avoid drinking alcohol and coffee, smoking and taking medications such as decongestants, diuretics and anti-anxiety drugs which reduce saliva flow allowing bacteria to proliferate.

- Sugary drinks, chewing gum and candy can leave a sugar residue that promotes rapid bacterial growth. Drinking during meals dilutes stomach acid needed for proper digestion.
- Foods which are a problem for you. Common bad breath culprits are strong cheeses, dairy, canned fish, processed meats, garlic, onions and curry spices.

Eat more:
- Green leafy vegetables for vitamins, kiwi, papaya and pineapple for digestive enzymes and other fruits and vegetables for dietary fiber.
- Yogurt or other probiotic foods that can aid digestion.
- Zinc-rich pumpkin seeds, oysters, or red meats.

Exercises:
Try any of the vigorous breath and voice exercises in Chapter 45. Then ask a friend or spouse if your breath has cleared.

Going to the Source:
None.

14 CHRONIC FATIGUE SYNDROME

When Helen was quite old and with more
energy left than strength, I asked her what her
idea of Heaven was. She replied, "Perpetual
activity without fatigue."
- Anonymous

In my opinion, one of the greatest disservices a physician can render a patient is to make a diagnosis of Chronic Fatigue Syndrome. There is no such entity. It is what honest doctors call a 'wastebasket diagnosis.' There are no specific abnormalities on physical exam and no specific laboratory tests that can identify this so-called disease. And of course, there is no specific treatment.

I understand the reasons why doctors are willing to make this diagnosis. Some are simply unable to admit that they don't know what is wrong with the patient. Others, in attempting to help, label the patient and in this way hope to organize their own thinking and that of the patient. Then advice and referrals can be made based on this (mis)diagnosis.

Most patients suffering the complaints of CFS are grateful when the doctor makes this diagnosis. 'At last I know what's wrong with me; now I can get the help I need.' I am sure that many patients thus diagnosed will be angry reading these words, but my task here is to bring clarity, not to further muddy the waters with garbage diagnoses.

Strong words, perhaps, but I have seen patients in effect become life-long cripples as a result of this and other wastebasket diagnoses. I am not blaming the victim here. I am in fact blaming the medical profession for their biggest deficit - they no longer listen to the patient.

To properly 'diagnose' a patient presenting with the complaints of fatigue, lassitude, aching muscles and joints and so on, an extensive history needs to be taken by the practitioner. This kind of medical history can take an experienced doctor at least an hour and a half to perform. It needs to be a bio-psycho-social-spiritual history, one that covers all aspects of the patient's current and past situations. And the doctor needs to listen with the ear of a physician and the sixth sense of a master detective. The answer, or the 'diagnosis' if you will, lies in the patient's words and how he speaks them. And the answer is a different one for each patient.

Since most suffering individuals will be unable to find a doctor who is willing or able to take that kind of history, I am offering here a self-cure approach to this problem. I understand fully that many patients diagnosed with CFS would prefer to retain the label and get what help they can from their doctor and CFS 'specialists.' But for the few who are willing to take another path, read on.

I can not offer you a treatment plan, even an alternative one, for a diagnosis that does not exist. What does exist are your symptoms. They are very real, not imagined, and are causing you great suffering. But it would also be folly for me to offer you advice and techniques for your specific symptoms. I have made that mistake in the past, resulting in temporary relief of one symptom while another flares up, needing attention, and so forth. For example, I have taught patients a vigorous breathing technique to counteract the mind-numbing fatigue. Or a meditation technique to clear the mind. Both with some success but always short-lived. The symptom complex quickly morphs into something requiring a different approach. Without a comprehensive approach, we wind up endlessly chasing symptoms around the body.

What is required is for you to become your own good doctor and great detective. Sit down with a pad and pen and a couple of hours to spare.

Close your eyes and in your mind go back to a time when you were free of symptoms. More than that, actually. To a time when you took your health for granted. Preferably to a time when you were healthy *and happy*. But if you were never happy, pay attention to that because it will come in handy. Even if you need to go back to childhood to find such a time, so be it.

Now, if you find that you have no memory of ever being happy (or at least content), I urge you to seek the help of a very experienced psychotherapist. You will not be able to figure this out on your own. The right therapist can, in the long run (and of necessity it will be long) help you more than your doctor can.

OK, let's say you have found that time in your life when you were healthy and happy. Now, write extensively about that time in your life: where you were living and with whom, what you were doing on a daily basis and with whom, and what your hopes and dreams were for the future. As you write, notice and make a note of the feelings and sensations that arise in your body and in addition, the feelings that you can recall from that period of your life. Take a break and give yourself time to digest what you have written and recalled.

At the next session, review what you have written. Then, move ahead in time to the next part of your history, your actual chronological progression. What did you do next in your life? Where did you live and with whom, etc. Take your time. Please do not rush this process. It might take weeks, but it's worth it.

So keep going in this vein until you come to a time when what you recall and what you are writing makes you uncomfortable. Do not look for obvious traumatic events. If traumatic events are part of your history- for example, the early death of a parent, a sudden uprooting of your home, violence done unto you – record them in your journal but make no assumptions. Instead, see how you feel as you write it down and then re-read it. As you then progress to the recollections of the next stage of your life, notice if the traumatic event is still haunting you. Often, it is not.

On the other hand, be careful not to gloss over some change in your relationships or circumstances by saying, well, it was hard but I got through it. Instead, as you are writing and reading, note the responses that arise in your body.

Sometimes a seemingly minor event can have a profound effect on your well-being, even though you 'think' it shouldn't have bothered you all that much.

For example, when I was in college, I had my heart set (notice the words I have chosen) on spending my junior year in France, studying at the Sorbonne. Through a fluke, that plan did not materialize. I went on with my studies and my life, but that was the year my symptoms began. It was not until years later that I realized that this non-event had changed the entire course of my life. It was then that I was able to recall that all my hopes and dreams for my future had been dashed, and I felt I had been betrayed by those close to me.

When, in your recollections and your writing, you reach that stage of your life history when your symptoms began, or you began to think of yourself as impaired or sick in some way, mark it well, so that you can easily find it again. Then continue with recording and observing of the next phase of your life. Chances are that from that point on, you will remember having either recurrent symptoms or a chronic condition that has persisted until the present.

If you have been lucky enough to identify this turning point in your life, what can you do about it? What relevance does it have to your present health issues? You think, so it happened, so what? Now I am stuck with this disease and I need help. It is at this point that you may be able to be your own best doctor.

Sometimes it is quite simple. A young man I knew years ago was suffering from a variety of somatic complaints. All he was able to manage was to go to work as an administrator each day and get through it, then come home exhausted. Using this historical process with him in my office, he discovered that he began to have serious symptoms soon after giving up his first love, performing rock music with a band he had put together. 'I gave it up because I had to get serious about my life, my wife and kids, that sort of thing,' he told me. At my urging, he dusted off his Gibson and began to play at home, alone, after work. His symptoms improved somewhat. I lost track of him but saw him on the street a couple of years later. He looked transformed. Indeed his life had been transformed. He had given up his boring job, put another band together, and was playing regularly at several venues. His wife had become the primary bread-winner, and although they were struggling financially, they were very happy, and healthy.

I have noticed this pattern frequently in creative people. For them, their art, or dance, or music or writing is an expression of who they are. When they are engaged in being creative, they experience a free flow of energy through their bodies. If this flow is interrupted for a long period, they tend to become ill.

I urge you, if you are a creative person who is currently ill with 'CFS,' dust off your 'instrument' and engage with it for a couple of hours each day, no matter how bad you feel or how busy your life is. Who knows where your life will go from there. Be fearless in your pursuit of what feels healing. In the long run others will benefit also.

I should add here that although I have had little experience with athletes, I suspect that having to give up a sport at which you have excelled may also be deleterious to your health. Good athletes are in 'flow' when they are at their best, and interrupting that flow surely can be sick-making.

I have chosen to include my observations on creativity and health in this section on Chronic Fatigue Syndrome, a non-disease. However, I have seen many patients experience an amelioration of symptoms from other diseases and conditions as well with this 'treatment.'

Sometimes it is not so simple. However, if you pay close attention to the process I have described above, and you find that turning point, know that therein lies the key to your getting better. For some of you, the quality of your relationships with others is the most important thing in your life, even though you may be hesitant to admit that. There may be deep disappointment and resentment regarding your relationship with your spouse or one of your parents, yet you have failed to bring that to light for fear of losing that person or of being 'unfair.' Yet it is more unfair for you to remain sick and become a burden on the other. If you risk speaking your truths, and you lose that special person, you will experience heartbreak. But you will recover from heartbreak after awhile. On the other hand, if you do nothing, your chronic fatigue will be life-long.

For others of you who are very goal-directed, it may be that a professional disappointment is at the heart of the onset of your disease process. Sometimes even a 'good opportunity for advancement' has been the wrong choice, for you. I have known several people who gave up working with their hands for a job with more pay who have suffered mightily for it. This too can be turned around, if we value good health over the acquisition of wealth and power.

If you want to recover from CFS, you must give up hope that some new piece of research will reveal the cause and therefore the definitive treatment for the condition. Viruses, parasites, toxins in the environment, genetic aberrations. The list goes on. Even if eventually a true cause and effect process is identified, there is probably little that can be done. On the other hand, remember that our bodies have an innate tendency to heal themselves, but to do so, our psyches (or souls, if you prefer) must also be engaged. Once again, I urge you to look for the answers within. You can do more for your health than your doctor can.

15 COUGH

*The ancient inhabitants of this island were less
troubled with coughs when they went naked,
and slept in caves and woods, than men now in
chambers and featherbeds.*
- Sir Thomas Browne

Cough is one of the most frequent presenting
complaints in the doctor's office and therefore merits
its own category. However, we should remember that
cough is a symptom and not a diagnosis. Just as pain is
an indication that something is wrong, so it is with
cough. Before instituting a treatment for symptom
relief, it is best to know the cause.

Cough is most frequently due to a minor illness or
condition, such as a viral respiratory infection, allergy or
dry air, but when the cough is persistent (i.e. longer
than a few weeks), serious disease should be ruled out.
*A visit to the doctor is indicated when the cough is persistent or
when it is accompanied by fever for more than a few days. If you
are coughing up blood or have shortness of breath, go immediately
to the doctor.*

The use of cough suppressants has never made sense to me, except perhaps at bedtime to ensure adequate rest for the day ahead. The cough is there for a reason – usually the body's attempt to get rid of an irritant in the respiratory tract – so to suppress that response is to invite a worsening of the underlying condition.

Self care of cough:

For cough due to asthma or allergies, see the remarks under those headings above.

For cough due to dry air: It is 'normal' to have a cough response to dry air in your home and it is easy to remedy. Buy an inexpensive humidistat to measure the level of moisture in your home. If the level is below 40%, it is important to add moisture to the air because the drying out of your respiratory passages renders you more susceptible to infectious disease. Room humidifiers are easily available and relatively inexpensive. I prefer these to central humidification (attached to your furnace) because they are more easily cleaned after use and less subject to contamination with mold and bacteria. If you keep the moisture level above 40%, you should notice a marked reduction in your cough.

For cough due to viral upper respiratory infections, drink lots of clear liquids and keep the moisture in your room high.

If you have a persistent cough *and your doctor has done a thorough evaluation* and has found no underlying pathology, consider the following self care approaches. However, if you do not get relief from them after a few weeks, get a second opinion regarding the etiology (cause) of your cough.

Nutritional:

A cough is the most common reason for visiting a primary care physician in the United States. Following the 7 Guidelines for Eating Well in Chapter 3 will reduce inflammation and help the body defend against and heal infections that cause coughing. Coughing serves a positive purpose to clear mucus. After a common cold or flu has cleared, a dry cough can persist for weeks. The repetition of coughing produces inflammation which produces discomfort, which in turn produces more coughing and so on. To naturally suppress a cough, take a teaspoon or two of honey before bedtime. Honey and lemon can be drunk alone or added to a tea made with soothing herbs such as eucalyptus leaf, fennel, ginger, horehound, licorice, marshmallow root, mint, mullein, slippery elm and thyme (which is also anti-bacterial). Coughs with a persisting cause (e.g. smoking, post-nasal drip, asthma, bronchitis or gastroesophageal reflux disease) should be treated by addressing the cause rather than simply suppressing the cough.

Get plenty of rest and eat immune boosting and anti-inflammatory foods rich in vitamins A, B and C (e.g. green leafy vegetables, berries, carrots and colorful fruits) along with immune boosting herbs (e.g. Echinacea), mushrooms (e.g. reishi, shiitake). It might be a good idea to take a break from nightshade vegetables (tomatoes, peppers, eggplant, potatoes) and to reduce the intake of sugar (sparingly use honey instead) as these can suppress the immune response in some people. Homemade chicken soup (made with stock, chicken, onions, sweet potatoes, parsnips, turnips, carrots, celery stems, parsley, salt and pepper) is at least as effective as over-the-counter medications and has a lot more nutrition. Foods high in omega-3 fatty acids are also generally anti-inflammatory and should help.

Avoid eating:
- Sugar and artificial sweeteners,
- Nightshade vegetables,
- Evidence shows that over the counter cough medications are no more effective than either honey or chicken soup.

Eat more:
- Green leafy vegetables, berries, carrots and other colorful fruits.
- Chicken soup, pastured turkey, liver, and eggs, wild salmon or tuna, bananas, avocado, Brazil nuts and molasses which are good sources of B vitamins and omega-3's.
- Honey (raw and local) and soothing herb teas.

Exercises:
Do breath exercise number 4 in Chapter 45, the Great Circle Breath, every morning as instructed. Also, sing loudly every day for a period of at least ten minutes.

Going to the Source:
Sit in a chair in the meditative posture and focus on your breathing, without attempting to control it in any way. If you have the urge to cough, let it come as much as it wants to, until you feel 'coughed out,' then return to an awareness of your breath. Keep this up for about 20 minutes once or twice a day. If this process is helpful, you can also use it for shorter periods

throughout the day when you have episodes of coughing.

Note: In my experience, cough is not often a nervous habit. When it is, a few sessions of psychotherapy should be helpful. Much more common is a nervous clearing of the throat. This occurs more frequently in children and should not be commented on by the parent. Instead, the source of the child's underlying anxiety should be determined and steps taken to remedy that.

16 DEPRESSION

For so your doctors hold it very meet,
Seeing too much sadness hath congealed your
blood
And melancholy is the nurse of frenzy.
Therefore they thought it good for you to hear
a play
And frame your mind to mirth and merriment,
Which bars a thousand harms and lengthens
life.
- Shakespeare, The Taming of the Shrew

Depression is another one of those conditions that is estimated to have a frequency of 20% in our population. Therefore, it is to be considered a life-style condition. It is the height of absurdity to regard one out of every five persons as having altered brain chemistry and therefore requiring treatment with prescription medication.

I do not wish to imply that there is no such thing as real depression. Any well-trained and experienced psychiatrist or clinical psychologist can recognize such a patient when they walk into his or her office. The seriously depressed patient has certain mental and physical characteristics that vary little from patient to patient and from day to day. These patients require intensive treatment with whatever methods the doctor has at his or her disposal. I do not know the incidence of this type of severe depression, but it is not common.

If you do not have this serious type of deep depression, but are told by your doctor that you will become that way unless you take anti-depressants, do not believe him. Chances are good that your bout of 'depression' will pass with no treatment whatsoever.

Most people who are labeled by the medical profession as being depressed are simply going through a period of feeling lousy as a result of things going wrong in their lives. I understand that if you are 'depressed' and are reading this, you will object to my trivializing your suffering with words like 'feeling lousy' and 'things going wrong.' If you prefer 'in the pits' or 'hopeless,' that's fine. Just please don't do yourself the disservice of calling yourself depressed, because these days you will be expected to take medication. That expectation will be held by your friends, family and your doctor and is very difficult to resist.

If you are now taking an anti-depressant and it is working for you and you want to continue taking it, the rest of this section is not for you. You can always return to these words if your meds are no longer helping or if you are experiencing unacceptable side-effects from the drugs.

OK, if you are feeling melancholy but don't want to take medication or you have tried the drugs and can't tolerate them, please continue reading. Before I get specific about self-care, let me answer a question which has probably been bugging you for some time: Why me? A lot of people go through a lot worse situations than mine and don't get depressed. Doesn't that mean there is something wrong with me?

If you ask that question of your doctor, he or she will probably tell you that it's because of your genetic make-up, which has resulted in your abnormal brain chemistry and that this needs to be corrected via psychopharmacology.

I can't prove to you that that is not true, nor can they point to research that says that it is true. It is just the current approach used by the medical profession. Time will tell, but you can't wait that long.

My answer to your question is this. It doesn't matter. If you are suffering from mild to moderate depression and do not wish to take anti-depressants, you have a couple of good choices, and actually I would recommend that you choose both of them. The first is to seek out a seasoned psychotherapist who believes what the research has shown: *That psychotherapy in mild to moderate cases of depression is just as effective as anti-depressant medication.* The second choice is self-care.

Nutritional:

Eating junk food can make you depressed. Unstable blood sugar levels and nutritional deficiencies associated with eating fast food worsen depression. Following the 7 Guidelines for Eating Well in Chapter 3 protects against depression. When feeling low, seek out the high levels of antioxidants in fruits and vegetables and the folate found in broccoli, cabbage, spinach, lentils and chickpeas. In addition, the omega-3 fatty acids found in pastured meat, wild fish and flaxseeds can be helpful.

If you're drinking diet soda – stop. Aspartame, the chemical sweetener in NutraSweet, Equal, Diet Coke, Diet Pepsi, and other drinks, has been shown to make depression worse in some people. Gradually reducing the amount of caffeine you consume by substituting water, decaf or herbal tea for caffeinated drinks might also help. Green tea, which has less caffeine than either black tea or coffee, helps calm mental worries, reduce stress hormones and balance neurotransmitter levels, all of which can reduce feelings of depression.

Comfort foods are literally foods that make us feel better based on a sense of nostalgia, indulgence or the specific physical comfort they provide. The best comfort foods are home made, and associated with positive emotional memories. There is evidence that eating these foods, in moderate amounts, actually helps the body cope with chronic stress and can help with depression. Ask yourself, "When I'm feeling low or tired and stressed or sick in bed, what food would I like a loved one (mom) to fix for me?" Some people like a hearty soup or fried chicken; others prefer macaroni and cheese, chocolate cake or toast with butter. Write down your list and arrange to have the ingredients to make these foods available. There is nothing wrong with a fattening comfort food if you make it a treat.

A special word about chocolate – dark chocolate (with a high cocoa content – at least 40%, but preferably 60%, 70% or even higher) can be particularly useful. About one ounce per day of dark chocolate can boost brain levels of endorphins and serotonin which can directly improve your mood. Dark chocolate is good for your blood pressure, lowers bad cholesterol, helps to prevent disease and improves both mood and immune function. Some of these benefits come from resveratrol, an antioxidant immune system booster also found in red wine. However I do not recommend drinking red wine for depression as alcohol is a depressant. Milk can interfere with the body's absorption of antioxidants, so don't substitute milk chocolate.

Some plants and herbs often help with depression including licorice, ginger, St. John's Wort, Siberian Ginseng, Damiana, and Ginko biloba as well as rose, sage, jasmine, lavender, sandalwood and orange. These can be found in over-the-counter herbal supplements or teas. Start by trying a cup of herbal tea with one or more of these ingredients in the morning or evening and see if you feel at all uplifted. Generally, what works for you is right.

It's difficult to prepare meals (or do anything for that matter) when depressed, but if you can push through your resistance, cooking can really help. Share meals and meal preparation with others when possible. Take the time to notice what you are eating and enjoy it and the process as much as possible. There is an old saying – 'when times get tough, start cooking.' I have found this to be true.

Avoid eating:
- Fast foods, junk foods, and sweet drinks as their food additives, trans fats and sweeteners may worsen depression.
- Caffeine and alcohol.

Eat more:
- Fruits and vegetables, especially berries, broccoli, cabbage, spinach, lentils and chickpeas.

- Better quality protein and fats including omega-3 fatty acids found in wild salmon, tuna, pastured meat and poultry, sardines, and flaxseed which are anti-inflammatory and help the body maintain proper neurotransmitter levels.
- Dark chocolate (about one ounce per day). This can boost brain levels of endorphins and serotonin which can directly improve your mood.
- Green tea which also balances mood and can be combined with other helpful herbs.

Exercises:

Conventional exercise: No need to get fancy or spend money, just walk. Every day, preferably in natural surroundings, walk at a good pace (three to four miles per hour) for at least two miles. This alone will make a big difference in your mental/physical state.

I am aware that one of the characteristics of being in the pits is that it is very hard to motivate yourself. I can not motivate you through the printed word any more than I have done so already. If you know of someone who is willing to walk with you and will not take no for an answer, enlist their aid.

Here is a technique that will help you to get started in the morning. If you are brave enough to do it, it will give you enough of a lift to get you out walking. The only equipment required for this technique is an adjustable shower head.

Take your regular morning shower. When you are finished, adjust the spray to be as concentrated as possible. Turn the water to very hot, but not scalding. Concentrate the spray on the area of your back between your shoulder blades. Keep this up for three minutes. Then turn the water to *very* cold and spray the same area for one minute. Then repeat this process for at least one more round, two if possible. Always end with cold. As you exit the shower, notice the change in your mood and/or energy level. If it is helping you as much as I think it will, make it a daily practice.

Breath and voice exercises: Do exercise numbers 3 and 5 in Chapter 45 every day.

Singing is very important here. Always start with a song that reflects what you are feeling at the moment. If you are feeling sad, down, sing that. If you do not know the tune and lyrics to a song that fits for you, make it up. Sing your sad words to your sad tune. Keep it up, getting as loud as you can, for at least ten minutes. A good place to do this is in the car on the way to work.

For some of you, dancing can be very helpful. Again, your dancing should reflect what you are feeling. Put on some music that fits for you at the moment, and dance your private dance to it for at least ten minutes.

If you are experiencing repetitive thoughts as part of your 'depression,' thoughts that recur over and over and seem to have a life of their own, here is an exercise that will give you relief from that symptom (which is called perseveration) and eventually eliminate it.

Stand in front of a mirror. Begin to talk in gibberish, using no 'real' words. Talk to the person in the mirror, letting the nonsense words flow *without thinking* of what you are saying. Use a lot of facial expression and hand gestures to get across to that person in the mirror. Keep this up for at least five minutes and do it twice a day.

Finally, be sure to spend at least three minutes a day laughing out loud. Your laughter does not need to be 'real' in order to be helpful. Just make the sound of Ha-ha-ha-ha-ha, loud and clear and keep it going. You can do this in bed when you first awake or even during your shower or while driving to work.

Going to the Source:

Meditation can be helpful during bouts of mild to moderate depression. I will describe the techniques that I have found most helpful. Please note that if you are *severely* depressed, do not attempt to meditate. It could result in a worsening of your condition.

Sit in a chair in the previously described meditative posture. Close your eyes and focus on your breathing, without attempting to change it in any way. After a few minutes, shift your attention to your body, letting your awareness roam through your body, so to speak. Pay attention to whatever feelings, sensations or symptoms arise.

If you are lucky enough to experience an emotional reaction as you sit, open yourself fully to it. It might be anger, or sadness, or even joy. Whatever it is, let it suffuse your body, breathe with it, let it get bigger. Sit with that emotional experience until it passes.

I say 'lucky' because, as you will recall, when we allow the free flow of energy and feeling through the body, this moves us in the direction of good health. Very often, a person's bout of 'depression' comes as a result of 'stuffing' his or her emotional response to a particular situation. This might start out as a conscious process, a clamping down on the feelings we are having (in order to avoid confrontation perhaps), but then becomes a chronic holding that we are no longer aware of. If we can retrieve that buried emotion and open ourselves to it, the depression will probably lift.

If your meditation makes you aware of nothing more than a generalized heaviness, lethargy, dullness throughout the body, try this visualization technique. Sit as erect as possible and breathe out fully three times. Then 'see' yourself leaping into the air, higher and higher until you are flying. Fly over your house and city into the surrounding countryside. Soar over lakes and woods and pastures. Try to keep the image of flying going for about three minutes, then bring yourself safely back to earth. Note if there are any changes in your bodily sensations.

On the other hand, if your meditation makes you aware of an internal agitation, a buzzing or vibratory sensation, you will need a different approach. Ask yourself (your body) what it needs to get relief, then wait for an answer. It might come in the form of an image, a sensation or a phrase. It may come and go so quickly that you will tend to dismiss it. Pay close attention and make no assumptions about what you will 'see' or 'hear.' If you are able to get the message from your body, then use your imagination to give yourself what you need. You may need to see and feel yourself being held and rocked in your mother's arms. If so, give that to yourself and give yourself over to whatever feelings might arise.

The approach just described can also be applied if you become aware of specific symptoms. Examples might be an aching in the chest, an emptiness or a craving in the belly, or a tension in your jaw. Ask your body what it needs and proceed from there.

A final note: If any of these techniques provide some relief, you may need to keep them up for weeks or months in order to get through your bout of 'depression.' Don't become discouraged. If you wish to speed up and enhance the process of healing, consider consulting a psychotherapist. This combination of self-care and psychotherapy, though time consuming, is well worth it. Not only will you avoid the hazards of taking psychopharmaceuticals, you will experience significant personal growth.

17 DERMATITIS

The power of making a correct diagnosis is the
key to all success in the treatment of skin
diseases; without this....therapeutics at once
cease to hold their proper position, and
become empirical.
- Louis A. Duhring

Dermatitis is not a diagnosis. It is a catch-all term referring to almost any condition of the skin, although it literally means inflammation of the skin. If you are told by your health care provider that you have 'dermatitis,' with no additional explanation, it probably means they don't know what is wrong.

A diagnosis of 'contact dermatitis' is usually good news. It simply means that your skin is reacting to something it has come in contact with. It might be a new laundry detergent or a chemical used in your workplace. Once you figure out what the offending substance is, the obvious cure is to eliminate contact with that item. It is not wise to use steroid ointments and creams or other skin preparations and at the same time continue contact with the substance that caused your rash.

Most other skin conditions are a reflection of some underlying dysfunction in the body. Whether it be a nutritional deficiency, an allergy, an auto-immune disorder or any other disease, it is important to arrive at a diagnosis before treatment is instituted. Most experienced dermatologists are helpful in this regard and I encourage you to consult with one of them. Once a diagnosis is made, treatment needs to be directed toward the underlying problem.

Please refer to the specific diagnostic categories for recommendations for self care of these underlying conditions.

Can dermatitis be due to unresolved emotional conflict? I had serious doubts about that possibility until an experience with one of my patients made it clear that the answer is a resounding yes. Elaine was a 30 year old medical secretary who had suffered from severe, disfiguring psoriasis of both legs for the past five years. She had been treated by dermatologists with almost no improvement. Even during the warmest months of the year, she had to wear long pants to spare herself embarrassment. She had sought my help to deal with depression related to sexual abuse as a child. As part of my work with Elaine, I had her perform the kicking exercise 3b described Chapter 47. At the next visit, she reported that doing that exercise at home on a daily basis had resulted in almost complete relief of her psoriasis. I was astounded, but of course suggested that she continue with the exercises as well as our psychotherapy sessions. She continued to improve and to my knowledge her skin condition remained resolved.

18 DIABETES

Man may be the captain of his fate, but he is
also the victim of his blood sugar.
- Wilfred G. Oakley

We will be dealing here only with Type 2 diabetes, the so-called adult onset type.

(Type 1 diabetes, known also as Juvenile Diabetes, needs to be expertly managed by specialists in the field, and while self-care methods can be helpful in preventing some of the long-term complications of the disease, even these should be monitored by a physician.)

In recent years there has been a marked increase in the incidence of diabetes, just as there has been with allergies and asthma. While the reason for the increase in the latter two conditions is arguable, it is clear that the frequency of diabetes is co-incident with the marked rise in obesity in our population. Obesity in turn is related to the consumption of grossly unhealthy foods, as well as an inactive life-style. It is relevant also that both obesity and diabetes occur with greater frequency in the poor and undereducated.

It is obvious that the epidemic of diabetes will only be curtailed when steps are taken to alter the life-style of those prone to the disease. Whether this is the role of the government or of individual citizens depends on one's political views. We can not deal with those kinds of ethical issues in a book on self-care.

In my opinion, the treatment of diabetes, especially in the early stages, is the same as the measures that should be taken to prevent the disease. I've heard doctors say, "you can't convince those people to exercise and eat healthy, so we just have to treat the condition as best we can." It is true that many people, especially obese people, are extremely resistant to dietary changes and are mostly unwilling to exercise. It is also true that an entire industry has grown up around that concept. A lot of people are making their living from the ravages of this disease and one wonders how motivated they could be to insist on life-style changes in their patients.

And then there is the issue of role-modeling. In the typical hospital-based treatment facility for diabetes (and many other chronic conditions), I have observed that a preponderance of the staff (clerks, technicians, LPNs and other 'physician extenders') are obese, and these are the people who have most contact with the patients.

Self cure of diabetes.

It is worth restating that these self cure methods will be most effective in the early stages of the disease.

Nutritional:

Diabetes type 2 is almost always entirely avoidable by following the 7 Guidelines for Eating Well in

Chapter 3, exercise and maintaining a healthy weight. Diabetes type 1 is much more manageable by following the same guidelines. If you already have diabetes (either type) and want to live as normally as possible with minimum medication, then you can modify the guidelines for eating well, eliminating grains, starchy vegetables (e.g. potatoes), legumes, as well as alcohol, sugars and juices from your diet. That means you'll still be eating 2/3 vegetables, but the remaining 1/3 on your plate will be made up primarily of protein and fat. It will not include extra carbs, except a limited amount of whole fruit with all the fiber nature provided to slow absorption of sugars. Non-starchy whole vegetables (e.g. spinach, kale, collards, asparagus, broccoli, cabbage, string beans, fennel, onions, leeks and celery) have plenty of carbohydrates to keep you healthy, but like whole fruits they are full of dietary fiber which slows its absorption into the blood stream.

Frequent small meals are superior to fewer large meals. It's best to prepare your own food, as packaged and processed food often contain unhealthy amounts of salt, sugar and other carbs. Be especially careful to avoid high-fructose corn syrup. When you begin to follow these dietary guidelines, be careful to review any diabetes medications with your physician to avoid lowering your blood sugar too much. If you aren't taking medications currently, then this diet may help you to avoid medications in the future. Your body will adapt itself to your new eating pattern and your health will improve naturally. As always, listen to your body and note any particular foods that cause you problems.

Certain herbs and spices are helpful in managing or avoiding diabetes. For example, chili peppers contain capsaicin, which works with insulin to reduce blood sugar and is a powerful antioxidant, whether dried, cooked or raw. Eating foods prepared with sea salt, cinnamon, fenugreek, and sea vegetables such as dulse, nori, wakame, kombu and hijiki help the body regulate blood sugar naturally. Brewer's yeast, liver, cheese, wheat germ, apples with the skin, spinach, oysters, carrots, and chicken are rich sources of the mineral chromium which significantly improves blood sugar metabolism and raises levels of HDL ("good cholesterol"). Zinc is also important and foods rich in zinc include fresh oysters, ginger root, lamb, pecans, peas, egg yolk, beef liver, lima beans, almonds, walnuts, sardines, and chicken.

Avoid eating:
- Processed and fast foods, sugar and artificial sweeteners, alcohol, and juices
- Grains, starchy vegetables, legumes.

Eat more:
- Non-starchy whole vegetables (2/3 of what's on your plate) raw, steamed or cooked in coconut oil, butter, or olive oil.
- Pastured meat, poultry, eggs and dairy, wild-caught fish, and a limited amount whole fruit. These should total about 1/3 of what's on your plate.

Exercise:
Walking is the easiest and the best. Here is a relatively painless method of getting started. Measure off one tenth of a mile in your neighborhood. A typical big city block is one twentieth of a mile, so two blocks would be one tenth. An easy way to measure is

watching the odometer in your car and noting the landmarks.

The first week, go out for a one tenth mile walk *twice a day*, rain or shine, hot or cold, no matter how tired you are. Cover the distance as fast as you can. The second week, add another tenth to each outing. By the time you reach week number 10, you will be walking two miles a day! That, along with your nutritional program, should be sufficient.

If you are unable to walk because of foot problems, enroll in a swimming program if one is available or go to a gym and ask for a non-weight bearing exercise program. Or if you are being treated in a multi-disciplinary diabetes clinic, ask the physical therapist for a series of non weight-bearing exercises you can do at home.

Going to the Source.

The following technique should be helpful to you in sticking to the nutritional program detailed above. Sit in a chair in the meditative posture. Close your eyes and focus your attention on your breathing. Feel the flow of air coming in and going out. Now concentrate on the exhalation, the flow of air going out of your lungs. See if you can make each out-breath last a little longer than the previous one. See if you can train yourself to breathe out continuously for a count of ten (seconds). When you have accomplished this, do it ten times. Then let your breathing return to its natural state. Now, sit quietly and turn your attention to the sensation of hunger or craving that you feel in your body. Do not try to rid yourself of this feeling. Simply sit and notice the feeling (whether it is constant or comes and goes) for ten minutes.

When you have done this 'exercise' faithfully for a couple of weeks, you may notice that the cravings are not so strong. Or, you may notice that despite the craving, you are stronger and do not have to give in to it. You will then be ready to eat the right foods in the right amounts to turn your diabetes around.

19 EARACHE

Most gentle Sleep! Two nights I wooed in
vain;
Thou wouldst not come to banish racking
pain:
For what is Sleep but Life in stone bound fast?
Oblivion of the Present, Future, Past."
- Francis Hard, After Two Nights of the Ear-
Ache, Weird Tales, October 1937.

Obviously earache is a symptom and not a diagnosis. I include it here because it is one of the most common complaints that bring people to the doctor. In children, it is *the* most common presenting complaint in a pediatrician's office. It is also one of the most over-treated conditions.

No pediatrician wants to risk not treating a full-blown ear infection with antibiotics. Untreated bacterial (as opposed to viral) infections in the middle ear can lead to serious complications such as meningitis (a potentially fatal condition) and rupture of the eardrum with subsequent permanent hearing loss. Hence, doctors tend to treat earaches with antibiotics even if there is substantial doubt in their minds as to whether it is bacterial in origin. Better safe than sorry, they say. What they don't say, of course, is that if they treat with antibiotics they cannot be sued for malpractice; whereas, if they opt for a watchful waiting approach and a complication occurs, they are vulnerable to a lawsuit. So it is a real dilemma for even the most conscientious practitioner.

Many children have recurrent bouts of earache due to a variety of reasons that have nothing to do with a bacterial infection. These children are overtreated with antibiotics frequently, which leads to problems which affect their long-term health. Oral antibiotics kill bacteria and this includes the normal and necessary bacteria that live in our intestines. This can lead to diarrhea, yeast infestation, allergies and, in my opinion, other chronic conditions. It can also lead to the development of antibiotic-resistant strains of bacteria which is a problem not only for the particular child but for others who come in contact with him.

If your child (or yourself) is suffering from a moderate to severe earache which lasts longer than one day and especially if accompanied by fever, see the doctor.

However, if you don't want to risk the complications of overtreatment, here is an approach which you can use with the doctor. Tell him or her that you don't want an antibiotic unless he is quite sure from the appearance of the eardrum that the condition is bacterial. He will say 'we can never be 100% sure,' which is true. Then request that he order a STAT (immediate) white blood cell count from the nearest laboratory. This takes only moments to perform and is not (or shouldn't be) expensive and gives the doctor significant additional information about whether the disease is bacterial. If the white count is normal, I would suggest a period of watchful waiting without treatment, provided that the same practitioner will be available to take your phone call over the next 48 hours. If so, you are quite safe in waiting. Then you can call the doctor if the problem does not subside or obviously if it gets worse.

This approach is safe only if you are assured of being able to contact the same doctor who has already seen the child. Otherwise, the risks of 'miscommunication' outweigh the risk of taking the antibiotic.

If the earache is *not* due to a bacterial infection and if there is no hearing loss, there are a variety of self-care methods that can be helpful, both for treatment and prevention.

Nutritional:

For relief of mild to moderate earache not associated with fever, instill a few drops of warm sesame or olive oil into the ear canal and leave in for about five minutes. When you get up the oil may harmlessly run out of the treated ear.

Exercise:

If the patient is an adult or a school-age, cooperative child, try this amusing and often effective exercise. Grab both ears with thumb and forefinger and pull the ears outward, away from the head. Holding this position, open the mouth as wide as you can and stick the tongue out as far as it will go. Now, make the sound 'aaaahhhh' as loud as you can and hold it a few seconds. Keep holding the position and making the sound for about two minutes. Repeat the exercise every hour or so throughout the day.

This exercise straightens the ear canal and helps to promote drainage of any fluid which may be 'stuck' in the middle ear, thus relieving pressure and pain. The ear pulling part of the exercise can be used with younger children, especially as a preventive measure in those kids who seem prone to frequent earaches.

20 ENDOMETRIOSIS

This condition is fairly common among patients seen in a Gynecology practice. No one seems to know why or how the lining of the uterus 'migrates' to other areas of the pelvis, attaching itself to the Fallopian tubes, ovaries, bladder and bowel and causing significant symptoms such as pain, infertility and dyspareunia (painful intercourse). The usual treatment of this condition is laparoscopic surgery, but the problem often recurs, sometimes necessitating hysterectomy.

I have seen this condition only a few times in my practice of mind/body medicine and certainly do not believe I have an answer to this problem. However, the experience I had with a couple of patients was so dramatic that it warrants recording here. Perhaps others will find it useful.

A young woman came to me because of anxiety but also reported that she was having great difficulty getting pregnant and was told by her gynecologist that she had endometriosis. She also suffered from pre-menstrual tension and dyspareunia. She carried a lot of tension throughout her body but this was particularly severe in the pelvis, where she was capable of only minimal movement. During the course of my treatment of her, I showed her a series of exercises designed to free up the pelvic muscles and bring more energy, feeling and movement into this area.

Within a year her pre-menstrual tension had abated and her pelvic pain markedly reduced. A few months later she became pregnant and subsequently delivered a healthy baby boy. She told her friends that I had 'gotten her pregnant.' Follow-up a few years later revealed that she had no further symptoms of endometriosis.

Her exercise routine consisted of the following. If you are suffering from endometriosis and feel that your pelvis is 'tight' or limited in motion (i.e. you are not much of a belly-dancer), it would be worth your while to try these exercises.

Energizing (Chapter 46, Exercise 2)

Kicking (Chapter 47, Exercise 3b)

Knee squeeze and release (Chapter 49, Exercise 4)

Abdominal rubbing (Chapter 49, Exercise 2)

Pelvic bounce (Chapter 49, Exercise 3)

21 FIBROMYALGIA

Physicians think they do a lot for a patient
when they give his disease a name.
- Immanuel Kant

This 'diagnosis', often applied to patients with chronic muscular pain, merits the same unkind words I used in the introduction to Chronic Fatigue Syndrome. It is a 'waste-basket' diagnosis, as any straight-talking physician will tell you. It is not useful to the patient because it sets up a series of assumptions and expectations that block a more creative, intuitive look at the suffering of the patient. And it invites treatment with a host of dangerous medications, often in combination, thus rendering them even more deadly.

If you have been diagnosed with this condition, or believe that Fibromyalgia is your problem, I urge you to read carefully the section on Chronic Fatigue Syndrome and to follow the procedure for self-care outlined there. If you prefer to go with an alternative approach, I would suggest finding a very experienced acupuncturist and, if possible, a body-oriented psychotherapist. These are your best options for getting over this devastating condition.

22 GINGIVITIS

DENTIST, n. A prestidigitator who, putting metal in your mouth, pulls coins out of your pocket.
- Ambrose Bierce, The Devil's Dictionary

Inflammation of the gums, with or without secondary infection, can be very unpleasant and potentially dangerous. It is usually considered to be caused by the build-up of plaque on the teeth beneath the gum line. Plaque, we are told by dentists, is secondary to poor oral hygiene and failure to have the teeth regularly cleaned by a dental hygienist. I include the condition here because in my limited experience, plaque and gingivitis can be prevented by some very simple self-care measures at home, thus avoiding the somewhat painful and expensive cleaning in the dentist's office.

Nutritional:

Following the 7 Guidelines for Eating Well in Chapter 3 will do a lot to prevent and even reverse gingivitis. Take particular care to limit alcohol and avoid sugars, soda, processed foods, baked goods, fruit juices and other carbs which saliva converts to sugar that feeds the bacteria causing gingivitis. Vegetables and fruits that crunch naturally help to clean your teeth and supply nutrients that fight the growth of harmful bacteria. Eating yogurt helps gingivitis by providing both protein and probiotics (helpful bacteria) which will displace some of the harmful bacteria causing your inflammation.

If you are suffering from gingivitis, a rinse of 1.5% solution of food grade hydrogen peroxide after brushing and flossing will kill harmful bacteria in the mouth. You should also stop using tobacco. Certain herbs and spices are helpful in managing or avoiding gingivitis. Neem and goldenseal are powerful anti-bacterial herbs which are included in some toothpastes. The folate in curry leaves also fights gingivitis. Chamomile, echinacea, rose hips, mint, hawthorn berries, cloves and caraway seeds are also anti-bacterial and anti-inflammatory. Try using them in cooking or herb teas. It is also helpful to eat an anti-inflammatory diet as described in Chapter 52.

Avoid eating:
- Processed and fast foods, quit smoking and limit alcohol.
- Sugars, soda, processed foods, baked goods, fruit juices and other carbs that promote unwanted bacterial growth.

Eat more:
- Green leafy vegetables, asparagus, peas, lima beans, almonds, walnuts, and pecans.

- Pastured meat, poultry, eggs and dairy, and wild-caught fish, shellfish, especially fresh oysters, egg yolk, sardines, beef liver, turkey, lamb and chicken.
- Whole fruit such as fresh pineapple, papaya, bananas.
- Ginger, chamomile, echinacea, rose hips, mint, hawthorn berries, cloves and caraway seeds which can also be helpful at reducing inflammation and infection.

Exercises:

In addition to brushing and flossing, I urge you to perform the following two preventive mouth treatments on a daily basis. In the morning, before eating, use your index or middle finger to massage your gums very methodically. Be fairly vigorous, spending at least 30 seconds in each quarter of your mouth, with emphasis on the area where the gum meets the teeth. This stimulation brings energy and blood flow into the gums and is especially important if your diet consists largely of soft foods. *Please note that this is a preventative measure and may not be appropriate if you already have gingivitis, especially if the gums are bleeding or infected – see your dentist.*

The second exercise I call 'salivary mouth wash,' and is useful as both a preventative measure and for treatment if the condition is not too severe. It is effective because the saliva contains enzymes which reduce unwanted bacteria and exert a healing effect on the mucosa. The exercise can be done when you are alone and do not need to talk for a few minutes, such as when you are driving or watching TV. Collect a mouthful of saliva by running your tongue around the inside of your mouth to stimulate salivary flow. Then swish the saliva around in your mouth as you would do with a mouthwash. Keep this up for at least three minutes. Finally, swallow the mouthful of saliva in small portions and notice the 'clean' sensation in your mouth.

Going to the Source:

This section is included because it is clear that in some cases gingivitis is yet another manifestation of stress. If you think this applies to you, pick any of the meditation exercises in Chapter 50 which you think might help you achieve the relaxation response and practice it daily.

23 GASTROINTESTINAL PROBLEMS

*That would be cool if you could eat a good
food with a bad food and the good food would
cover for the bad food when it got to your
stomach. Like you could eat a carrot with an
onion ring and they would travel down to your
stomach, then they would get there, and the
carrot would say, 'It's cool, he's with me.'*
- Mitch Hedberg

Also known as the 'gut,' the G-I tract actually
extends from mouth to anus. While the mouth belongs
to the dentists, the rest of the gut is in the purview of
physicians.

Technological advances have made it possible for
specialists in the field to have an 'up close and personal'
look at every inch of your gastrointestinal tract, and
they seem to have a fascination for doing just that. The
esophagus, the stomach, the duodenum, the small and
large intestines and the rectum can all be "scoped."

Most of these specialists spend a lot more time
scoping than they do talking with their patients. I

suspect they are aware that the medical history is ninety percent of the diagnosis, but this task is left to the less experienced members of the team (nurses, NP's, PA's) or to a printed history form. The history of a patient with gastrointestinal complaints is more often than not a study of human nature, and I find these histories fascinating. It's a lot like playing detective. And since most of what ails these folks occurs as a result of lifestyle choices, it is also rewarding to solve the 'mystery,' and to be able to make recommendations which, if followed, will result in a cure.

The good news about scoping and other high-tech interventions in the gut is that it enables gastroenterologists to detect serious, life-threatening disease early. Mostly we are talking about cancer – esophageal, gastric, colon – which all seem to be on the rise in recent decades. Unfortunately, these early intervention procedures have not been proven to save lives. Depending on how statistics are interpreted, sometimes early treatment seems to prolong life if proper treatment is instituted.

If you are concerned about cancer anywhere in your gastrointestinal tract, see your doctor right away.

There are numerous conditions that affect the gut and many of them are different manifestations of the same underlying condition. For the sake of clarity, let us begin at the top and move to the bottom, the same way our digestive process works.

Difficulty Swallowing:

In children, this problem is almost always 'emotional,' and is fairly common in anxious school-age kids. It is transient and will resolve after a short time if the parents do not over-react. The child should be reassured that this happens to lots of kids and is nothing to worry about. Further, the parents should advise the child to eat whatever he can manage to swallow and not to worry that he will starve. *In the unlikely occurrence that the child swallows and then the food comes back up, it is time to see the doctor.* This may be an indication that there is actual obstruction of the esophagus or that the emotional problem is severe enough to warrant intervention.

In adults, the same caveat holds. *If the food comes back up into your mouth or if the swallowing difficulty is constant, see your doctor right away.*

Fortunately, difficulty swallowing is usually 'functional;' that is, it is a symptom that has no underlying pathology – no obstruction and no ulceration of the esophagus. Doctors often diagnose this problem as due to 'spasms' of the esophagus, and indeed this may be the case, but the real issue is why do these spasms occur. No one seems to know.

One of my patients, whom we shall call Diane, developed an intermittent swallowing difficulty while she was in therapy with me for severe anxiety. At my request, she kept careful track of when the symptoms occurred. We discovered a clear pattern: when she had strong feelings towards one of her friends or family members which she felt she could not express, the symptom became so severe for a few days that she actually lost weight. Gradually she learned to express those feelings in a manner that was not destructive to the relationship. Since then the symptom occurs only on rare occasion and lasts only a few hours.

Exercises:

Upper Abdominal Rubbing: Lie on your back with a small pillow under your head. Relax for a moment or two then begin rubbing as follows. Use the heel of your hand against the bare skin of your belly. Begin with the right hand, placing it on the upper right corner of your belly, just underneath the rib cage. Using firm pressure, sweep the heel of the hand slowly across the upper abdomen to the upper left corner. Do this in the same direction 36 times. Now switch hands. Use the left hand to rub from the upper left to the upper right corners, again 36 times. Rest for a minute, keeping the belly soft, before getting up. Do this as often as necessary. You may find it beneficial to do this before each meal.

Going to the Source:

In my experience, you are much more likely to develop a swallowing problem if there is tension at meal-time. If you are rushing through the meal in order to get somewhere on time or if there is fighting and arguing at the table, you are clearly not relaxed at this time. The digestive process, starting with the enzymes in the mouth, is impaired when you are tense and angry, or fearful. If the enzymes that are necessary for digestion are not flowing, it makes sense that the body will want to reject the intake of food. Think of an animal. If your dog is disturbed when he is about to eat, he will back off the food and deal with the problem at hand and not return to the food until he feels 'safe.' Follow his example.

One way you can relax before a meal without having to solve all your worldly problems is to do a brief meditation. Follow the instructions in Chapter 5 to induce a relaxation response and then take a couple of minutes to scan your body, especially your throat, chest and belly, for signs of tight, tense muscles and then consciously relax each segment until the area feels 'open,' and ready to receive food. It is difficult to do this at first, but with practice you will find that you can do this in less than a minute, anytime, anywhere, without anyone noticing what you are doing.

Gastro-Esophageal Reflux Disorder (GERD)

This condition has become so 'popular' in our culture that it has earned its own acronym. It used to be called 'acid indigestion,' and would be cured, we were told, by taking 'Tums for the tummy.' Interestingly, the old advertisements for Tums clearly referred to our 'over-indulgence' in food and drink as the cause of the problem and indeed that seemed to be the case for most of us. Now, however, it is considered a disease state requiring not an adjustment of our eating habits but necessitating a prescription medication.

I find it sad that most people with this problem seem to be reassured when they are told by their doctor that they have 'GERD,' an actual disease. I guess they are relieved that they don't have to spend time worrying about the quality of what they are putting in their stomachs or about the functional state of the body that is receiving that food. And, lucky for them, the pills really do seem to 'work;' that is, they do relieve the symptoms of GERD.

For those of you who like to think outside the box and in fact don't like to be put into a labeled box at all, consider the following. If you are eating food that your body seems to have trouble digesting, it makes more sense to take a hard look at that food and/or at why your body can't handle it. If we mask the symptoms with a cute little pill, what are we doing to ourselves in the long run? Questions like this intrigue me and probably you as well if you are reading this book.

If you are not consuming a healthy diet, this may be the source of your reflux problem. Please refer back to Chapter 3: Intake for information about healthy foods. If you already eat nutritious food but still suffer from reflux, it may be your style of eating that is the culprit. Rushed meals, tension at the table, eating too late in the evening (especially if you go to bed shortly after dinner), can all contribute to a reflux problem. As mentioned above under Difficulty Swallowing, a simple meditation technique can prepare you for a relaxing meal and may well eliminate the source of the reflux. In addition, the following self-care methods will address the issues underlying GERD.

Nutritional:

GERD is 100% preventable and largely reversible by maintaining proper nutrition, eating habits and weight. Start by following the 7 Guidelines for Eating Well in Chapter 3. The most effective tactics for preventing GERD are weight loss, eliminating tobacco and avoiding excessive alcohol intake. To further prevent GERD, don't drink with meals – particularly cold liquids, eat smaller meals, especially at dinner and avoid eating within two to three hours before bedtime. A cup of miso broth before a meal can aid digestion.

Pay attention to which foods and beverages cause you problems and avoid them. Many people find that GERD symptoms are brought on by alcohol, coffee, carbonated beverages, processed or fast foods, chocolate, citrus fruits and juices, tomatoes, tomato sauce, spicy or fatty foods, full-fat dairy products, peppermint or spearmint, chewing gum and hard candy. Sometimes more subtle food intolerances cause GERD, for example dairy and gluten. Try eliminating them from your diet one at a time to see if it helps.

Ginger is one of the most highly effective foods for soothing acid reflux. Ginger relaxes the muscles in the esophagus, aids digestion, and acts as an anti-inflammatory, antimicrobial and analgesic. Fresh ginger root can be added to recipes or made into a tea. Pickled (sushi) ginger can be added as an accompaniment to any meal. If your esophagus is not inflamed, then black pepper or long pepper (pippali) freshly ground onto food also helps stimulate digestion.

If your esophagus is irritated and inflamed, you will also want to avoid acidic foods such as citrus fruits and juices, ketchup and other tomato products, mustard, pepper, vinegar, hot peppers, beer, wine and soda. A soothing tea (not with meals) can help reduce the inflammation and promote healing. Green tea, ginger, fennel, Indian gooseberry (amla), chamomile, meadowsweet, barberry, dandelion root, licorice, marshmallow root and slippery elm are good ingredients. Slippery elm and marshmallow root also contain mucilage which can form a protective gel in the stomach and lower esophagus, protecting it from acid. Try aloe vera juice in your tea, prepared by scraping the fresh gel from inside the stalk of the plant into a blender with some tea. This will reduce inflammation and help heal the lower esophageal sphincter that prevents reflux.

Avoid eating:
- Too much, especially close to bedtime.

- Processed and fast foods which are problematic. Also stop using tobacco and limit alcohol, especially beer and wine.
- Coffee, carbonated beverages, chocolate, citrus fruits and juices, tomatoes, tomato sauce, spicy or fatty foods, full-fat dairy products, peppermint or spearmint, chewing gum, and hard candy which can all contribute to GERD.
- Acidic foods if your esophagus is irritated, such as citrus fruits and juices, ketchup and other tomato products, mustard, pepper, vinegar, hot peppers, beer, wine and soda
- Foods which cause you problems (dairy and gluten are common culprits).

Eat more:
- Green leafy vegetables.
- Smaller meals, especially dinner, and hours before bedtime.
- Healing teas between meals including green tea, ginger, fennel, Indian gooseberry (amla), chamomile, meadowsweet, barberry, dandelion root, licorice, marshmallow root, slippery elm and aloe vera juice.

Exercises:
The patients I have seen with reflux problems all have one thing in common – they have a significant degree of tension in the diaphragm. I can not say with certainty that this is the sole cause of the reflux, but it does make sense given our anatomy. It is the diaphragm that separates our chest (thoracic cavity) from our abdominal cavity. It is at that location where the

esophagus, which is in the chest, enters into the stomach and at that juncture there is a functional 'valve' which is supposed to keep food from coming back up from the stomach into the esophagus.

I have noticed that when the diaphragm is tense, the upper abdominal muscles (the ones just below your ribs) are also tense. With all these powerful muscles exerting pressure on the stomach, does it not seem reasonable that the 'valve' might not hold, giving rise to a reflux problem. In any case, those patients of mine who have successfully learned to relax these muscles have seen a marked reduction in their reflux symptoms.

To achieve relaxation of the diaphragm and upper abdominal muscles, try the following exercises:

a. Upper Abdominal Rubbing as described under Difficulty Swallowing.

b. Abdominal Breathing as described in Chapter 4.

It is important to note that neither of these exercises should be done on a full stomach. Try to find time to do them twice daily when the stomach is completely empty.

Going to the source:

As noted above, a brief meditation focused on the chest and abdomen before each meal should be very helpful.

If you have the time for a deeper psychophysiologic awareness of the problem, please try the following. After eliciting the relaxation response, turn your attention to your solar plexus, which is the area just below your sternum (breastbone) in the midline of your body. Gently place one or both hands on this area and continue to breathe easily *through your mouth with your jaw relaxed*. Now ask the question, what do you need to feel safe enough to relax and open? Then wait for an answer from your solar plexus. Have no expectations about what you may 'hear' or what images you may have or what you may feel in your body. Simply pay attention to what comes and to what emotions, if any, are evoked by those messages from your body.

Ulcers of the Stomach or Duodenum:

Thanks to the discovery that ulcers are associated with the bacterium H.Pylori, conventional treatment of this problem has become simple and usually effective. There is usually no need for a lot of high-tech procedures to make the diagnosis as the symptoms are fairly characteristic: An upper abdominal pain, often experienced as a burning sensation, and most severe when the stomach is empty. It is usually temporarily relieved by eating.

Consult your doctor if you think you may have an ulcer because the complications of an untreated ulcer can be life-threatening bleeding or perforation.

If you find that you require long-term treatment with prescription medication in order to keep you free of ulcer pain, or if ulcers are a recurrent problem for you, you may want to consider an alternative path. In my opinion, chronicity or recurrence indicates an imbalance in your gastrointestinal tract, secondary to either nutritional inadequacy or psychological issues, or perhaps both.

Nutritional:

Follow the 7 Guidelines for Eating Well in Chapter 3 to establish a strong nutritional basis. Proper nutrition is the single most important factor in preventing and healing ulcers. A common home remedy, frequent glasses of milk, actually may make ulcers worse over time. Milk neutralizes acid in the stomach, reducing pain, but the digestive system reacts to this by producing more acid. My personal experience with ulcer and gastritis is that eating good quality sauerkraut quickly relieves the symptoms. Another way to get quick relief is juicing fresh cabbage and drinking half a cup up to 3 times a day. Add yogurt with live cultures to your diet to balance your intestinal flora. You may find goat or sheep's milk yogurt to be less inclined to irritate than cow's milk.

Cut down or cut out the common culprits of ulcers including non-steroidal anti-inflammatory drugs (NSAIDs, e.g. ibuprofen), smoking, aspirin, alcohol, coffee (even decaf!), tea, chocolate, fried foods and excess salt. Drink pure water between meals and try eating six smaller meals instead of three larger ones. It is not necessary to eat a completely bland diet. Make a note of spices and other foods which cause problems and avoid these. If a certain spice does not cause issues, then it is fine to use it. While you are at it, make sure to note other foods that cause problems as food allergies can contribute to problems with ulcers.

Avoid eating:
- NSAIDs, aspirin, alcohol, coffee, chocolate,
- Junk, fast, and fried foods,
- Food allergens or spices that cause problems.

Eat more:
- Frequent, small meals,
- Yogurt with live cultures,
- Good quality sauerkraut or fresh cabbage juice.

Exercises:
Belly rubbing at least three times a day.

Going to the Source:
Ulcers have been associated with H.Pylori and elimination of the bacteria 'cures' the ulcer. But this does not mean that stress has no role in the development of the condition. Nowadays most people are under stress, so why do relatively few develop ulcers?

The effects of stress on the body varies with the constitutional make up of the individual experiencing that stress. Some are prone to respiratory problems, others to musculo-skeletal problems, still others to gastrointestinal problems and so forth. This is one reason why not everyone under stress gets ulcers.

The development of bodily ailments as a result of stress is called somatization. It has become very clear to me that those of us who do not fully experience our emotions and do not find an appropriate way to express those emotions are subject to physical symptoms which can lead to actual disease states. In the words of the Woody Allen character in the movie *Manhattan*, " I don't get angry; I grow a tumor instead."

What can you do if you are one of those people, like me, who have a tendency to somatisize? The approach has to be a general one. Otherwise, you will be chasing symptoms around your body for the rest of your life. An ulcer, then perhaps lower back pain. A few years later tension headaches or chest pain or TMJ. You get the idea.

To alleviate your current set of symptoms and to prevent development of others, I suggest the following. One, learn meditation and practice it faithfully on a daily basis. Two, practice expressive exercises, lots of them, on a daily basis for as many years as it takes (usually at least two years). Three, consider some long-term (two to three years) psychotherapy with an experienced body-centered psychotherapist.

This one-two-three approach takes commitment and often entails a significant change in life-style. However, you will be rewarded with improved mental and physical health for the rest of your life.

Crohn's Disease and Ulcerative Colitis (Inflammatory Bowel Disease):

These devastating diseases of the small and large intestines often become manifest during the teens or early adulthood and are usually life-long problems. It is thought that there is a dysfunction of the immune system that lines the digestive tract which results in inflammation and destruction of tissue. This in turn causes debilitating symptoms and serious complications.

Physicians readily admit that there is no medical cure for these diseases and that sometimes surgery is necessary to remove diseased segments of the bowel. This however does not prevent the disease from flaring-up in other segments.

The medications that are available for use in treatment of Inflammatory Bowel Disease are numerous and all of them seem to have very serious side effects. Their use is justified because the relief of debilitating symptoms that they may provide is sometimes worth the risk.

I have had only minimal experience with patients with these conditions (which does not surprise me because the disease begins relatively early in life and is so severe that patients get locked into the conventional medical approach). Therefore I do not feel competent to offer suggestions for self-care.

However, I would like to offer an observation. It is well established that almost all patients go through long periods (months or years) of remission from the disease. These remissions are clearly not always related to treatment and therefore occur spontaneously. It makes a lot of sense to me for doctors and patients alike to delve deeply into what is going on in the patient's life during the periods of remission compared to the times when flare-ups occur. I would suspect that there are psychological stressors that precede the recurrence of the disease process. Remember, everyone responds to stress in their own unique way and it is clear that the gastrointestinal tract is a frequent target.

Despite my lack of concrete experience in this area, I would like to enthusiastically recommend meditation as a complementary intervention no matter what course of treatment the patient has chosen. I know of no other process that reduces 'inner turmoil' as effectively as the practice of daily meditation.

IBS - Irritable Bowel Syndrome

This is another one of those acronymic hodgepodges that is said to occur in 15% of the population, clearly making it a life-style disease. Physicians call it a functional disease of the bowel because no pathology can be demonstrated. Once again, labeling of patients in this manner is not beneficial to their well-being because it limits creative analysis of the problem. The symptoms are real enough (though usually transient) and include abdominal discomfort, bloating, excessive gas, diarrhea (mucousy at times) or constipation.

Physicians have established criteria for making the diagnosis, as they have with Fibromyalgia. Alas, these criteria are based on the subjective symptoms of the patient and are therefore hopelessly flawed. There are no objective physical or laboratory abnormalities that can make the diagnosis. There is also no specific treatment.

The most frequently overlooked 'real' disease in patients who have this set of bowel symptoms is Celiac Disease. Patients are often tested for cancer and for Inflammatory Bowel Disease when they present with vague intestinal symptoms, but all too often the doctor does not think of testing for Celiac Disease.

If you have symptoms that sound like Irritable Bowel Syndrome, make sure your doctor orders tests to rule out Celiac Disease.

In terms of Self-Care, there is much that you can do to eliminate the symptoms of Irritable Bowel.

Nutritional:

The best way to improve irritable bowel is through changes in eating habits. Start by following the 7 Guidelines for Eating Well in Chapter 3. This diet is high in helpful fiber, vitamins, minerals and enzymes and low in processed foods and typical gut irritants, so irritable bowel may resolve itself after a few weeks. IBS is not a specific disease, so no one diet will work for everyone. Keep a food journal, make note of what works for you and avoid foods make you feel worse or trigger cramping, gas, diarrhea or constipation. It can also help to pay attention to how you eat. Put your fork or spoon down, and chew each bite fully before picking the cutlery up again. This will slow down the process and allow your saliva to begin the digestive process. Also try to eliminate stress and distractions while eating so that you can pay attention to the process and enjoy it more.

Avoid fast food, alcohol, coffee (even decaf), carbonated drinks, tobacco, artificial sweeteners or sugar substitutes, foods and drinks high in sugar, especially soda, candy, cookies and other packaged sweets, artificial fats (e.g. Olestra, Crisco and other trans fats) until you know whether they are causing issues or not. Deep fried foods and bacon or sausage and other high fat foods may trigger irritation in some. For others, fruit juice, dried fruit, dairy (e.g. milk, cheese, ice cream, butter, sour cream), coconut milk or egg yolks may be the culprit. Some find poultry skin and dark meat or red meat a problem, while others find grains (especially wheat, rye, barley and baked goods containing gluten) to be irritating.

If intestinal gas is an issue, then determine which foods cause it and avoid them. Typical culprits are beans, broccoli, brussels sprouts, cabbage, cauliflower, apples, dried peas, lentils, chives, peppers, artichoke, green beans, leeks, onions, cilantro, celery, carrots, raisins, nuts, bananas, apricots, prunes, wheat germ, pretzels, and bagels). Certain medicines are associated with IBS too.

Raw vegetables can cause problems for some including cucumber and lettuce in salads. The following vegetables can cause problems even when cooked: broccoli, brussel sprouts, cabbage, cauliflower, corn, kohlrabi, leeks, onions, bell peppers, pimentos, radishes, rutabaga, sauerkraut, scallions, shallots, turnips, and chili peppers. Dried peas, beans, and lentils (the bean group) can cause problems, and some fruits such as apples with peels, avocadoes, cantaloupe, honeydew melon, prunes, and watermelon. Other foods and drinks that may cause trouble include beer, seeds (sesame, poppy, sunflower and flaxseed), hard-boiled eggs, carbonated drinks, nuts, wheat germ, and popcorn. Since many of these foods have a lot of nutritional value, it's worth the effort to determine if they are or are not a cause of your problems.

Coffee (including decaf) contains an enzyme that irritates the entire digestive tract and can trigger abdominal spasms, diarrhea, and a very unpleasant sense of urgency. Coffee is also highly acidic, and contains caffeine which can aggravate IBS as well as GERD. If you've been drinking decaf, you can quit cold turkey without caffeine withdrawal headaches. Try Teeccino (a blend of herbs, nuts, fruits and grains that are roasted, ground and brewed just like coffee), decaf Chai (an Indian spiced-tea drink), or a helpful herbal tea of digestive aids peppermint, fennel, chamomile, anise, and especially ginger. Peppermint eases IBS by relaxing smooth muscles in the intestines, but don't take it if you are also experiencing reflux, as it also relaxes the lower esophageal sphincter. Similarly chocolate is beneficial for irritable bowel but could make GERD worse.

Artificial sweeteners can cause gastrointestinal side effects, particularly sorbitol, but also saccharine, Equal / aspartame / NutraSweet, Splenda / sucralose, xylitol, and malitol. Splenda is a laboratory altered molecule of sugar that passes through the gut without being digested, causing irritation. The same is true of other artificial sweeteners for some people. If that is true for you, use real sugar – sparingly and make it a treat.

Eating several smaller meals during the day, rather than three large ones, may help. Peeling and seeding fruits and veggies will remove the toughest insoluble fiber altogether. Chopping, cooking, and pureeing will mechanically break down the insoluble fiber in fruits and vegetables. Soak nuts overnight before eating to soften them. Fiber may also decrease bloating, pain, and other symptoms of IBS. The healthiest soluble fiber foods are root veggies (sweet potatoes, pumpkin, beets, rutabagas, carrots, etc.), ground flaxseeds, fresh fruits (berries, mangoes, bananas, apples, pears, peaches and apricots) as well as avocados. All may be tolerated better when cooked. The live cultures found in yogurt are helpful and better tolerated than other dairy products. If you are not lactose intolerant, then eat an organic yogurt without added stabilizers, thickeners, fruit or sweeteners.

Avoid eating:
- Too much at one meal.
- Processed and fast foods, stop using tobacco and limit alcohol, especially beer and wine.
- Coffee, carbonated beverages, and
- Any other foods which cause problems.

Eat more:
- Frequent small meals,
- Root vegetables and other sources of soluble fiber,
- Water and healing teas between meals including ginger, fennel, chamomile, and anise. Peppermint as well unless reflux is also a problem.

Exercises:
    a. Abdominal rubbing (Chapter 49, Exercise 2).
    b. Belly pumping (Chapter 50)
    c. Expressive Exercises (try any of the exercises in Chapter 47)

Going to the Source:

Many patients respond to a nutritional approach to this problem (see above) but there are others whose symptoms are clearly related to psychological distress. If you fall into the latter group, consider the following.

You may be a person who tries to take all things with equanimity. You think of yourself as calm and not easily ruffled. Yet you have these pesky bowel symptoms that are unpleasant and at times embarrassing. Why? The answer lies within.

Sit in a comfortable chair in a meditative pose (Chapter 5). Relax but do not meditate. Instead, think of a recent experience that was upsetting. I choose the word 'upsetting' because it is the word patients most frequently use to avoid saying that they were enraged or grief-stricken over a particular situation. It is a neutral word, one that keeps you from experiencing your real emotions.

So, re-play that upsetting experience in your mind and notice what somatic sensations arise in your body. Try out the words rage, grief, longing, and loneliness to see if any of them fit with what you are feeling. To the extent that you can experience the genuine emotion, your bowel symptoms will subside (on rare occasion, the suppressed emotion is excitement, which some patients have been taught is a no-no).

Hopefully, this technique will work for you. *If not, please consider therapy with a body-oriented psychotherapist to deal with your symptoms.*

Hemorrhoids

People do not like to talk about their anus or their bowel movements. I suspect there are a lot of folks who have hemorrhoids and struggle to deal with it themselves. I include the condition in this book because my own personal experience may be helpful to those of you suffering from this problem.

Prevention is important here as it is with most of the disorders we are considering. If your bowel movements are normal and you do not strain during evacuation, you probably will not develop hemorrhoids. Some people who are *not* constipated still exert pressure while defecating because they are in a hurry or because of a habit learned during childhood. The urge to defecate will occur naturally if you wait for it and when it comes, one needs only to relax and await the passage of the stool. You can learn to do this if you are willing to take the time. Your body will teach you. It is important NOT to sit on the toilet until you get the urge, because that position tends to inhibit the urge. Practice softening the belly and the pelvic floor and occupy your mind with some relaxing task while waiting.

A very helpful technique for women with 'sluggish' bowels was invented by a friend of mine with a sophisticated knowledge of female anatomy. It is based on the fact that the posterior (rear) wall of the vagina lies next to the rectum. To promote movement of the stool, insert a thumb into the vagina and stimulate the back wall of the vagina, gently assisting the stool in its passage through the anus.

What is a normal bowel movement? Doctors have always accepted any formed stool as within normal limits, so it might be better to ask, what constitutes a *healthy* bowel movement. In my opinion it is a stool that is formed but soft, bulky, of large diameter and voluminous. This indicates a complete evacuation of the contents of the sigmoid colon and rectum. In fact, after passing such a bowel movement, you will feel a refreshing emptiness in the lower abdomen. Healthy bowel movements depend on consuming a healthy diet (see section on nutrition) and on having a 'stress-free bowel' (see section on Irritable Bowel Syndrome).

If you already have hemorrhoids, try the following. First, correct your diet and avoid any straining at stool. Second, use *very* cold 'sitz' baths for three minutes twice a day. A proper sitz bath is a small tub in which you can immerse your pelvic area up to the belly button while the rest of you remains warm and dry, including your lower legs and feet. These sitz baths not only tend to shrink the hemorrhoid, but also tend to 'tonify' the entire pelvis. Third, use Preparation H liberally. I find this time-tested product (I believe it has been on the market virtually unchanged for over 60 years) very effective.

24 HEADACHES AND MIGRAINE

In headaches and in worry
Vaguely life leaks away,
And Time will have his fancy
To-morrow or to-day.
- W. H. Auden

Obviously, headache is a symptom and not a diagnosis. *Recurrent, severe headaches require a diagnosis in order to rule out life-threatening pathology. Your doctor can order tests to make sure you do not have a brain tumor, an aneurysm, a hematoma or another source of increased intra-cranial pressure.* These serious conditions are often treatable thanks to advances in high tech medicine in recent decades.

Once serious pathology has been ruled out, you are usually left with a diagnosis of either 'Migraines' or Tension Headaches. It can be very difficult for even experienced medical practitioners to separate out those two types of headaches, since the diagnoses are based on a constellation of symptoms rather than on physical exam or laboratory tests.

The classic symptoms of migraine (aura, unilateral pain, visual disturbances, photophobia, cold hands and feet, nausea) would seem to indicate a disturbance in the sympathetic/parasympathetic nervous system. This is a poorly understood and under-researched aspect of the nervous system, but it is clear that stress results in considerable imbalance in this so-called autonomic nervous system. It is also known that certain foods and chemicals can cause this imbalance and migraine sufferers usually know which items can precipitate an attack.

It is also clear that both acupuncture and meditation can help immensely in restoring balance to the autonomic nervous system. Despite the lack of definitive research linking these two disciplines to amelioration of migraine, I would urge migraine sufferers to try both of them. Both processes are completely safe and offer a wise alternative to conventional prescription medications usually used to prevent and abort migraine attacks.

If you feel that your headaches are most likely Tension Headaches and serious pathology has been ruled out (see above), please try the following self-care approach.

Nutritional:

Eating well and avoiding possible triggers can have a major impact – decreasing the frequency, severity and duration of headaches. Common headache triggers include smoking tobacco, drinking alcohol, dehydration, eating at irregular times, not getting enough sleep, additives in processed foods, artificial sweeteners, aged cheese, cured meats, smoked fish, red wine, beer, fermented food, yeast in freshly baked bread or cake and chocolate. Keep a food journal to determine if any of these are causing difficulty for you. Do not skip breakfast, lunch or dinner and avoid spiking your blood sugar by including protein and fiber in each meal. Headache can be brought on by dehydration, so drink water between meals.

Magnesium is essential for the normal functioning of muscles, blood vessels and brain chemistry and levels are often low in chronic headache sufferers. This nutrient is consumed in everyday activity, especially during menstruation and when drinking alcohol. Rather than taking supplements, try eating magnesium rich foods like leafy greens, wild seafood, nuts, seeds, pumpkin, bananas or avocados. Organic produce tends to have more magnesium as conventional fertilizer typically does not include this essential nutrient. Foods rich in vitamin B2 (riboflavin), coenzyme Q10 and ALA (alpha lipoic acid) are also helpful. Some important foods are green leafy vegetables, bananas, fresh oysters, ginger root, lamb, pecans, peas, egg yolk, beef liver, lima beans, almonds, walnuts, sardines, turkey and chicken.

Aspartame (Nutrasweet, Equal) and Sucralose (Splenda) can be headache triggers. Avoid these and use Stevia, raw honey, 100% pure maple syrup or xylitol. Check labels to avoid inadvertently ingesting aspartame or sucralose in yogurt or other prepared foods. MSG (monosodium glutamate – common in Chinese food) is another additive to avoid. The relationship between caffeine and headaches is complex. Caffeine can relieve headaches if the body is not habituated to it. Two to three cups of coffee per day on a regular basis can increase headaches. Even one cup of coffee on a daily basis can worsen headaches in some people. If you experience "caffeine withdrawal" or headache after skipping your usual coffee, then you're probably drinking too much every day. Substitute coffee with herb tea, especially with ginger, valerian root, feverfew, or butterbur.

Avoid eating:
- Processed and fast foods.
- Your trigger foods.
- MSG or artificial sweeteners such as Nutrisweet or Splenda.

Eat more:
- Green leafy vegetables, asparagus, peas, lima beans, almonds, walnuts, and pecans, pumpkin seeds.
- Pastured meat, poultry, eggs and dairy, and wild-caught fish, shellfish, especially fresh oysters, egg yolk, sardines, beef liver, turkey, lamb and chicken.
- Whole fruit such as bananas. Teas with ginger root and valerian root.

Exercises:

The exercises suggested here work best when done early in the course of the headache. Once you have a full-blown tension headache (or migraine) that has persisted for a few hours, nothing is likely to work except sleep, deep meditation (with focus on the pain) or strong medication.

Head Lift: This requires another pair of hands. You can easily train a spouse, a friend or even a co-worker to help with this exercise.

You, the sufferer, lie on the carpeted floor or a very firm mat. Bend your knees so that your feet are flat on the floor. Relax your entire body as much as possible and remain passive while your helper works on you. That means *do not help* him or her.

The helper sits or kneels on the floor behind your head and cradles your head in both hands, overlapping his fingers at the base of your skull. He then very slowly and gradually lifts your head from the floor while reminding you not to help him lift. He keeps lifting very gradually until your chin comes down toward your chest. How far one can go is dependant on the flexibility in the neck. Signal your helper when he has lifted far enough.

As your helper is lifting your head, continue to breathe freely, emphasizing the exhalation. The helper holds your head in the flexed position for just a few seconds and then gradually lets it down to the floor. Repeat the process once or twice more, then remain resting on the floor for a full minute before getting up.

Isometric exercise: Sit very straight in a chair. Make fists with both hands and press the fists into your forehead, exerting pressure against your head while your head presses back into your fists. There is no movement. Hold this position while you open your mouth wide, stick out your tongue as far as possible and exhale noisily through your mouth. Hold the position for about 15 seconds. Then switch your hands to the back of your head and repeat the same process. When you release the pressure of your fists, do it slowly and gradually. Repeat the whole process two or three times, then sit quietly in the chair for a full minute.

Voice exercise number 5 in Chapter 45.

As an alternative to these exercises, if you are able to, cry/sob deeply for several minutes until it feels finished. If the sobbing is uninhibited, you will experience complete relief. If you are holding back, your headache may worsen.

Going to the Source:

Tension headaches occur, as the name implies, as a result of tension in the muscles of the head and neck. This tension often involves the muscles of the face and scalp as well as the large muscles at the back of the neck and upper back. Why do these muscles get so tense? Are you trying to keep from losing your head?

Pick a time when you are free of headache, or perhaps very early in its course. Sit quietly in a chair, breathe out fully several times and try to 'feel' the tension in your neck and head. Turn your attention to what is going on in your life at present. If you 'lost your head,' what would it look like? Would you shout and scream at someone or would you break down crying? Would you 'bite off someone's head' if you let loose of the tension in your jaw? "See" yourself acting out in a way that would feel satisfying to you.

I want to be perfectly clear. It is not necessary for you to act out against anyone either verbally or physically in order to get relief from your headache. What is important is that you become aware of the feelings that your muscles are protecting you from experiencing, and that you let those feelings flow through your body, without judgment.

In general, the more you can be aware of the feelings you are having as you go through your day, the less likely you are to have headaches.

As a general measure, ten to twenty minutes of meditation each day will eventually lessen your tendency to have headaches. Choose any of the meditative procedures outlined in Chapter 50.

25 HEART DISEASE

People get heart disease for lots of reasons. If
someone said, 'What's the most important
thing I can do to protect my heart health?' my
first answers would be, 'Don't smoke, get
exercise and eat a sensible diet.' But
somewhere on the list would be, 'Pay attention
to your relationships.'
- Dr. Tim Smith, University of Utah professor
of psychology
EMOTION, n. A prostrating disease caused by
a determination of the heart to the head. It is
sometimes accompanied by a copious
discharge of hydrated chloride of sodium from
the eyes.
- Ambrose Bierce

This section is for those of you who have already
been diagnosed with heart disease. If you are unsure
about your diagnosis, please first read the section on
Angina (Chapter 8). We are using the term heart disease
here as synonymous with coronary artery disease. While
there are other forms of heart disease ultimately leading
to heart failure, they are relatively rare and will not be

discussed here. These include, among others, congenital heart disease, cardiomyopathies, and heart valve pathology. These conditions require expert conventional medical and surgical care. I know of no effective self-cure strategies for these problems.

Coronary Artery Disease (CAD) is somewhat less common than it used to be, probably due to public awareness of the importance of good diet and exercise to heart health, and to a reduction in cigarette smoking in our country in recent decades. What is disturbing is the apparent increase in the number of men and women having heart attacks at an appallingly young age. It is no longer shocking to hear of someone in their 40's or even 30's suffering a heart attack.

When a young person who is obese and perhaps already suffering with diabetes or 'metabolic syndrome,' I am not surprised when they succumb to a heart attack. What does shock me still is when I hear about a heart attack in a young man or woman who lives a relatively healthy life style (regular exercise, good diet). When I discuss this with my doctor friends, they usually agree that it's probably because of our current fast-paced life-style, including the intense pressure to make money, leaving little time for relaxation and pleasure. I am not satisfied with this explanation. After all, nearly every young person these days is subject to the same stressors at work and home and bombarded with information overload, yet relatively few have heart attacks. I ask myself, what distinguishes these people from the others. Why them?

I have a theory about this which is completely without scientific corroboration. I present it here because if even one person feels that it fits for him or her, and makes the changes necessary to save their own heart (and life) it will have been worth it.

I think the young people who are subject to CAD and heart attacks are the ones who are too good, too fair and reasonable, too pleasant in their dealings with others. At work and at home, they are seen as nice guys, who rarely express negativity. Yet we know that when we are young, our passions run high and our feelings are strong. Maybe not as 'out of control' as when we were teenagers, but that energy is still coursing through our veins. If we have 'learned' to be reasonable and measured in our responses to all those around us – the inept clerk at the check-out counter, the unfair boss, our spouses, our ill-behaved children and dogs – we may be setting ourselves up for a heart attack.

When our behavior is so out of synch with what we are feeling deep inside, I believe this is a dangerous situation. Think for a moment about what you have to do in your body in order to hold back the strong feelings that come up during the course of each day. If you carefully observe someone who is not keeping such a tight rein on their emotions, you will notice that as the feelings begin to surface, the person breathes more heavily and becomes somewhat flushed. Soon they might break down crying or start shouting and gesticulating with their hands. This is normal human behavior, a release that is useful so that further honest dialog can continue. Of course the risk is that it might escalate to physical acting-out if the confrontation continues, but in my opinion it is worth the risk. Why?

Because what you have to do to suppress those perfectly normal feelings is, basically, to control your breathing. You control your breathing by constricting the muscles of your jaw, throat, chest and belly. Keep doing this long enough and often enough and it becomes a chronic state, in which you become unaware that you are feeling anything at all, setting you up for all kinds of health problems, including a heart attack.

Maybe what I am saying makes sense to you, and maybe you have not reached that state where you are unaware of any feelings, but on the other hand you believe that your daily life at work and/or at home is such that you can not safely express any emotions. Is there anything that you can do to get the release necessary to prevent a dangerous medical condition from developing? Yes, there is. Please read on.

Basically, there are two options for release: one private, one public. The private option you've seen in movies many times. You go to a safe place, your car or a room where no one can see or hear you, and you let yourself go – cry, scream, shout, kick, pound, throw things – until you feel the release. Then go back to your meeting and act like a so-called normal person.

The public options can also save your life. You are in a board room with other employees and the boss. Some jerk is saying something that denigrates your work or imputes your character and you'd like to leap-up and strangle him. But you have to sit quietly and look neutral and, incredibly, interested in what he is saying. What will save you is to use your breath and your imagination. Breathe out very slowly through your mouth, making it last as long as you can. Immediately take another breath and exhale again. If you are worried someone will notice you, do it behind your hand. At the same time, you can also picture yourself saying and doing exactly what would make you feel better. Beat the idiot to a bloody pulp in your mind, over and over if necessary.

At home, you can be a bit more direct. Let your spouse and your children see the early signs of your distress. Flushing and breathing heavily and perhaps tearing up indicate to them that you are upset. You can also say 'I'm getting really angry.' This approach is so much more effective with kids than a tight-lipped, cold reprimand or sending them to 'time-out.' It also teaches them that having normal human emotions is just that, NORMAL.

Let us return to the self-care of heart disease. Your coronary arteries are blocked and you are at risk for a coronary thrombosis (heart attack). Is there anything you can do beyond the surgical approaches of stents or coronary bypass procedures on the one hand or the conventional medical approach of multiple prescription medications on the other.

A few years ago, the 'alternative' methods of managing heart disease seemed to be getting a lot of press, especially the work of Dr. Dean Ornish on reversing heart disease. The research was clear. Heart disease could be effectively reversed with diligent attention to diet, exercise and stress-reduction via yoga and meditation. I am assuming that this approach did not catch-on with the public for a couple of reasons. It didn't make anyone a lot of money and it does take a lot of time on the part of the patient. It also is not very glamorous or dramatic compared with open-heart surgery.

For those of you who are more interested in long term good health and prevention of serious illness, and specifically methods to keep your heart healthy, I offer the following self-care methods. These are, admittedly, basically the same as the Ornish method with a bit more emphasis on dealing with feelings.

Nutritional:

It is clinically proven that heart disease can be prevented and even reversed by significant changes in diet and lifestyle. Follow the 7 Guidelines for Eating Well in Chapter 3, quit smoking, limit alcohol, and maintain a healthy weight. These steps along with exercise and stress reduction will prevent heart disease in the majority of people.

If one already has symptoms of heart disease, then it is a very good idea to follow a well-researched diet such as *Dr. Dean Ornish's Program for Reversing Heart Disease.* This diet consists of fruits, vegetables, whole grains, and legumes in unlimited quantities and excludes all meat and dairy, except egg whites, nonfat milk and nonfat yogurt. Caffeine is eliminated from the diet and sugar, salt, and alcohol are reduced. Take care to soak grains in water overnight. Nutritional supplements with folic acid, vitamin C, vitamin E, vitamin B12, fish oil, flaxseed oil, and selenium are included in the Ornish program, but these nutrients can be obtained by eating whole foods.

Fish (wild caught) such as halibut, salmon, cod, snapper, sole and trout as well as herring, mackerel, anchovies, sardines, and oysters are superior to fish oil gel caps as sources omega-3 fatty acids, but will need to be consumed in limited quantities to stay in line with the Ornish program's severe limitation of dietary fat. Freshly ground flaxseeds can be added to recipes instead of taking flaxseed oil gel caps. Wild fish and flaxseeds are also rich in selenium, vitamin E and vitamin B12.

Inflammation can also contribute to heart disease, so eating anti-inflammatory foods or the strict anti-inflammatory diet suggested in Chapter 52 is a good option. Foods high in omega-3 essential fatty acids have a very powerful anti-inflammatory effect. These include cold water oily fish (particularly wild salmon), walnuts, flax seeds, and pumpkin seeds. Extra virgin olive oil and natural coconut oil will also reduce inflammation and reduce the risk of developing heart disease. Ginger, turmeric (the main ingredient in yellow curry powder), green tea (decaffeinated) and red onions are also anti-inflammatory. Ginger can act as a blood thinner, so take care with its use if taking a blood-thinning medication (even aspirin).

Avoid eating:
- Processed and fast foods.
- Excessive fat, sugar and salt.
- Caffeine

Eat more:
- Green leafy vegetables (e.g. spinach, chard, kale, collards, dandelion greens), as
- Fruits and vegetables rich in vitamin C, E, B12, folate and selenium, especially berries.
- Wild-caught fish and fresh-ground flaxseeds.
- Ginger, turmeric, green-tea and red onions.

Exercise:
Conventional exercise: Please see the comments in Chapter 4 for advice on this type of exercise.

Other types of exercise for the prevention of heart disease and for facilitation of healing of coronary artery disease should all address one goal: *softening of the thoracic cage (the chest)*. If the chest wall is soft and moves freely, the 'heart will have room to breathe.'

Chances are you have no idea whether your chest is rigid or soft. The easiest way to find out is to visit an experienced massage therapist. By observation and touch, he or she will be able to tell you and to help you soften your chest (if necessary) with hands-on techniques. If you have been protecting your heart for years, it will be somewhat frightening when your chest begins to open up. However, nothing bad will happen to you. It is in fact useful to experience the fear and sadness that led you to 'wall off' your heart in the first place. If the feelings are overwhelming, do not hesitate to seek psychotherapy. Once again, I would suggest a body-oriented psychotherapist if you can find one.

You are not likely to be able to soften your chest on your own, but you can and should do a number of exercises to keep the chest open once the therapist has begun to work with you. If you don't do some work on your own, chances are your chest will remain tight except for a few hours following the therapy.

The following are the best self-care exercises to do to keep the chest soft.

Using a large exercise ball, place your chest on the ball and let your head, arms, lower torso and legs just hang loosely. Feel the ball holding you. Now let your breath out long and slow, preferably using a low moan to do so. Breathe out fully and hold it out for two seconds, then let the air back into your chest. Breathe out again and repeat the whole procedure about ten times. Each time, try to let your chest collapse into the ball more and more with each breath.

Sing a lot of sad songs, loud and clear and with great (even exaggerated) feeling. Songs of heart break. Feel your heart breaking. Cry (sob) if you can and let the tears flow until they stop naturally.

If you have young children, let them walk on your chest and back with bare feet. Do not resist the contact. Breathe out fully.

Do the mad man laugh exercise in Chapter 47 every day for at least five minutes.

Going to the Source:

You may have read in the popular press that getting angry increases your chances of having a heart attack. This well-meaning advice is misguided, based on inadequate understanding of how our feelings work. Becoming angry, or sad, or excited and so forth is part of being human. When our emotions flow freely though our bodies we are more alive and our health is enhanced.

On the other hand, being an angry person is not conducive to health. The word hostile fits better here. If most of the time you are seething, bristling with hostility, or on the edge of rage, you are certainly a candidate for heart disease. It is even worse (for you) if you try to present a calm, cool and collected face to the world. *If this description fits for you, you can save your life by seeing a good psychotherapist.* You can also do any of the anger-releasing exercises in Chapter 47.

Meditation on opening the heart (see advice above re softening the chest): Sit in a comfortable chair in the meditative pose. Close your eyes and breathe out fully three times. Bring into your mind the image of someone you love or have loved very deeply (it can even be a beloved pet). Feel the presence of that being in the room with you and let your love flow to them. Keep this up until you can feel your heart opening to that person. It may take only a few seconds. If the opening sensation does not happen within a minute or two, let go of trying and simply sit quietly and notice the thoughts that come into your mind. Do not create any thoughts, just let them 'pop up' into your head and observe your body's reaction to the thoughts. Stay with this process for at least ten minutes then slowly come out of the meditation.

26 HYPERTENSION

" ...I had a very difficult time...persuading my
colleagues that stress could be a contributor to
high blood pressure..."
- Herbert Benson, MD

High blood pressure has become so rampant in our culture that it must be considered a disease of life-style. Often people do not know they have hypertension until they visit a doctor for some other reason. In other words, they have no symptoms of elevated blood pressure. Of course, once the problem is discovered, both patient and practitioner are eager to do something about it. The patient is usually advised to get more exercise and reduce their salt intake but the mainstay of hypertension treatment is medication. Doctors routinely prescribe these drugs and patients take them unquestioningly. Not one of the many drugs prescribed for high blood pressure is without side effects, some of which are potentially dangerous, especially when used in combination with other medications.

Since the incidence of this condition is so high in our culture, one would think that a lot of attention would be paid to finding the underlying causes and to discovering ways to prevent the problem from developing. Sadly, no significant research money is directed toward those goals. The research is all about finding newer, more effective drugs. And the sad part of that is that the newer medications are proving no more effective than the older, less toxic ones.

I still recall the first patient I saw with hypertension when I began my practice of mind/body medicine three decades ago. He was a 35 year old administrator at an insurance company, a high-stress position which he handled effortlessly. However, at a routine physical he was discovered to have moderate hypertension. Before beginning the medication prescribed by his doctor, he sought my help. A careful history revealed that he was happy and effective at work and at home. We were both puzzled as to why he had developed this condition. I taught him a meditative technique and suggested he get some regular exercise, but after several weeks there seemed to be no improvement. He was discouraged and resigned himself to starting on the medication. On a hunch, I asked him what kinds of things brought joy into his life. On reflection, he realized that he was no longer doing the thing that in the past had given him the most pleasure: basketball. With my encouragement, he dropped his 'work-out' routine at the gym and began playing basketball with a 'pick-up' team several times a week. A couple of weeks later his blood pressure returned to normal and stayed that way without medication.

It is rare these days to find a patient who wants to have a serious discussion about the underlying causes of their elevated blood pressure, even among people who are educated and have some interest in living a healthy life-style. Nevertheless, I will put out my ideas about the self-care of hypertension.

First of all, one should consider what really constitutes an elevated blood pressure. Doctors have, of course, clear guidelines for the parameters of mild, moderate and severe hypertension. No one, including myself, believes that severely elevated blood pressure should go untreated. The risk for stroke or heart attack is too high. And patients with severe hypertension should be carefully evaluated for treatable underlying conditions which might be causing the problem, such as certain types of kidney disease and rare types of tumors.

Regardless of how the problem is discovered, if you have SEVERE hypertension, seek medical help as soon as possible.

It is another story, in my opinion, when it comes to evaluation and treatment of mild to moderate hypertension. No one is even certain that those levels constitute a threat to one's life, but such patients are usually medicated on the basis of the theory 'better safe than sorry.' That is, the blood pressure could rise to dangerous levels without the doctor knowing it and the patient can't be trusted to monitor his own levels. And of course there is the usual consideration of 'standard of care,' which means the tests, procedures and treatments generally followed by physicians in that specialty. The doctor cannot be sued if he or she has prescribed medication for your mild or moderately elevated blood pressure in a manner consistent with the standard of care.

Well, there is another path to be taken if the practitioner and the patient are willing to spend some time. First, the significance of the elevated pressure can be evaluated in the following manner. The patient needs to find someone who is skilled at taking blood pressures[5]. This is usually quite easy as most of know someone who is an LPN, EMT or another type of paramedical worker. The blood pressure is taken, with the patient lying down and relaxed, at least three times a week at random times of day for a minimum of a month. The worker records the results in a notebook but the patient is not told of the results. At the end of the month, the patient and doctor look at the notebook.

If the record shows that the blood pressure is variable from time to time, ranging from normal to mildly (or even at times moderately) elevated, this in my opinion does not warrant treatment with anti-hypertension medication. You should simply follow a life-style to prevent significant hypertension from developing, and should return every few months for follow-up.

On the other hand, if the record shows a consistent or recurring elevation into the moderate or severe ranges, then medical evaluation and possible treatment are indicated.

Diet, exercise and meditation are the mainstays of the prevention of hypertension and the treatment of mildly elevated blood pressure. This is the same protocol suggested for heart disease and several other life-style conditions. We often say that such conditions are 'stress-related,' and indeed that seems to be the case.

I have been curious for decades why some people respond to stress by developing coronary artery disease,

---

[5] In this case, I do not recommend self-recording of blood pressure using a home monitoring device, nor recruiting a family member to help. There is a need to eliminate variables which might affect the results in one way or another.

others hypertension, still others arthritis and so forth. It is easy to blame it all on one's genetic make-up, but I believe it is much more complicated than that. I believe it has a lot to do with how we handle our feelings. My experience has been that those persons who are fully aware of what they are feeling most of the time and are generally expressive, are much less likely to develop any of these conditions. But those of us who are out of touch with our emotions and rarely express how we feel are subject to one or more of these stress-related illnesses. Which ones we will develop and why remains a mystery to me.

Self-cure of hypertension:

The research is quite clear. The regular practice of meditation is just as effective as medication in lowering blood pressure in patients with mild to moderate hypertension. If you want to avoid the risks of taking anti-hypertensive drugs, start meditating right away. Please see the section on meditation (Chapter 50) to select a method that fits for you.

The other self-cure interventions, including nutrition, are the same as those listed for Heart Disease in Chapter 25. Eating grapefruit has an immediate effect on blood pressure in most people, so much so that it is prohibited for people that are on pharmaceutical blood pressure medication.

27 IMPOTENCE

What is it men in women do require?
The lineaments of Gratified Desire.
What is it women do in men require?
The lineaments of Gratified Desire.
- William Blake

In the male of the species, Impotence is now referred to as Erectile Dysfunction. ED is the politically correct term, used in polite company. It has been foisted on us by the pharmaceutical companies through the media. "Impotence" sounds like a problem, which it is. "Erectile Dysfunction" makes it sound like a disease (which it is not) needing treatment with a new class of drugs promising to bring romance back into our lives.

Does anyone honestly believe that a man can ingest a pill which will dissolve in the gut, be taken up by the blood stream, and go directly to the penis? The drug gets into all the organs in your body. These medications are new, but you can be sure that over the course of the next decade, reports of serious and perhaps life-threatening complications will be legion.

If it is a 'disease,' then it has to have a cause, which indeed it does. The underlying causes of impotence are psychological (eg, rage), medical (eg, diabetes), or drug-induced (eg, anti-hypertensives, psychotropics). My guess would be that prescription medications account for the majority of impotency problems in young and middle aged men. Do you really want to take another medication to counter-act the side-effects of your already risky combination of pharmaceuticals?

In my opinion, the only sensible course is to address the underlying causes of your impotency. If you have psychological issues, see a therapist; if you have medical conditions, get the best treatment available. And if you are on certain medications that you feel are interfering with your ability to maintain an erection (or for that matter, even your desire for sexual intimacy), see if your doctor can suggest an alternative to the drugs you are now taking.

Impotence in a woman is a much more complex situation. Unlike the male, end organ response in a woman is not easily 'measured," so it is difficult to say what exactly constitutes impotency. A better term is 'lack of sexual desire.' If we define it this way, then the underlying causes are the same as those outlined above for the male and need to be addressed in the same manner. For additional information on lack of desire in women, please see Chapter 29 – Intercourse Pain.

If all this sounds gloomy and discouraging, take heart. There are certain exercises and techniques you can use to enhance the flow of sexual energy though your body. These methods may work for you even if you have one of more of the underlying conditions mentioned above. They will certainly work if you have addressed your medical and psychological issues and have reduced or eliminated prescription medications.

Nutritional:

Following the 7 Guidelines for Eating Well in Chapter 3, eliminating tobacco, limiting alcohol and caffeine, and maintaining a healthy weight will help most men to avoid or reverse impotence. Excess body fat produces hormones that can disrupt erectile function. Alcohol depresses nerve impulses to the penis, while caffeine is a vasoconstrictor, reducing blood flow to the penis. Avoid trans fats and excess salt and sugar in refined, processed or junk foods.

Increase consumption of food rich in antioxidants, B vitamins, zinc, iron and selenium. These nutrients improve blood flow to the arteries that supply the erectile tissue of the penis. Richly pigmented berries (e.g. blackberries, black currants, blueberries, elderberries, raspberries, cherries, boysenberries, red/black grapes), pumpkin seeds, garlic, green leafy vegetables, walnuts, turkey and shellfish (especially oysters) are rich in these nutrients. Also make sure to get enough healthy protein and fats by eating pastured meat, coconut and extra virgin olive oil, wild cold-water fish (especially salmon, tuna, sardines, halibut, and mackerel). Liver from pasture-raised animals is an excellent source of iron.

If your impotence is occasional, keep a food journal and try to identify trigger foods. Eliminating these may solve the problem. Drink plenty of water between meals to keep the body properly hydrated. Herbal teas containing asian (panax) ginseng, saw palmetto, damiana, ginkgo biloba, muira puama, lubo, hu-chiang or yohimbe bark can also be helpful.

Avoid eating:
- Alcohol and caffeine,
- Processed, fast and junk foods.

Eat more:
- Richly colored berries, green leafy vegetables (e.g. spinach, chard, kale, collards, dandelion greens),
- Oysters, pumpkin seeds, garlic, walnuts,
- Pastured meat, liver and wild-caught fish,
- Helpful herb teas of ginseng, saw palmetto, gingko biloba and others.

Exercises:

Please see the special section on sexual exercises (Chapter 49) and follow the ones that seem to work for you.

Going to the Source:

Indirectly, meditation may help you overcome impotency. The twice a day practice of eliciting the relaxation response (Chapter 5) acts as an antidote to the ravages of stress on your body, bringing you back into equilibrium. When this happens, even your hormonal balance tends to normalize, and you may note a return of sexual desire.

You can also use the power of your imagination to 'jump-start' your sexual desire. This works best if used in conjunction with sexual exercises. When you are in a relaxed state, and breathing freely, allow yourself to imagine the situations that used to bring you to a state of sexual arousal. It is very important in this regard not to judge yourself. Images may arise which, if acted out, would not be socially acceptable. As long as you do not act them out, there is no problem. Erotic images used for your own arousal do not harm anyone else, and there is no shame in having them.

Another important point is this. If you begin to feel aroused and with that notice a concomitant restriction of your breath and/or a tightening of your musculature (especially in the pelvis), at this point you should stop. Try to relax the muscles and open your breathing while you are using imagery and doing the sexual exercises. If you are unable to do this after several attempts, please consider body-oriented psychotherapy. Restriction of the breath and tension in your muscles will seriously interfere with your ability to experience full sexual arousal and release.

A word about aging and sexuality in men: Many older men, even those in good general health, notice a decline in sexual desire. Many assume that this is just a normal part of aging and that there is nothing you can do about it. Indeed, nothing needs be done about it and some men do not miss that part of their life. But if you are an older man who longs for more sexual vibrancy, read on.

To restore your sexual energy, try most of the sexual exercises in Chapter 49. I would strongly urge you not to skip the self-massage routine described there or, as an alternative, schedule sessions with a massage therapist focused on stimulation of the skin.

If this approach does not seem to be working after a week or two, you might want to consider the approach advocated by practitioners of traditional Chinese medicine. Their view is that each time a man ejaculates, he loses some of his 'essence,' which cannot be fully restored. Therefore, as he gets older, the frequency of ejaculation should be markedly reduced. They suggest continued frequent sexual activity (alone or with a partner), but stopping short of ejaculation. According to Chinese medicine, by the time a man is in his seventies, he should not ejaculate more than a couple of times a year.

At first this retention of semen will feel like an 'incomplete' experience, that you have been deprived of something special. But as you learn to focus more and more on the pleasurable erotic sensations during sexual activity rather than the 'release,' you will not feel deprived and will enjoy the sensations of being sexually alive every day.

28 INSOMNIA

Sleep that knits up the ravell'd sleave of care,
The death of each day's life, sore labour's
bath,
Balm of hurt minds, great nature's second
course,
Chief nourisher in life's feast.
- Wm. Shakespeare, Macbeth

Almost every one of us experiences a bad night's sleep at sometime in our lives, perhaps due to jet lag, worry or even excitement. We grumble and complain, but know that when the situation resolves, we will sleep well again.

Many people have gone through periods in their lives when loss of sleep is more frequent and severe. Usually there is underlying stress, such as divorce, job loss, or chronic illness. Here the insomnia is a symptom and merits symptomatic relief by the use of over the counter or prescription medications. As long as these episodes are short-lived, I see no harm in the short-term use of such drugs. In order to cope effectively with these very real stressful situations, adequate sleep is necessary. If prescription medications are useful to you but you find that after a few days or weeks that they are no longer effective, try limiting yourself to an every-other-day routine. That way you will not build up tolerance and the side effects will be minimized.

Some individuals do not get a good night's sleep because certain life-style habits interfere. Examples of this are legion: excess alcohol consumption, eating a big meal before bedtime, watching stimulating TV programs, late night internet use, disregarding the cues our body gives us when we need to sleep (yawning, drowsiness, lethargy). The 'cure' for this type of insomnia is obvious: change the behaviors. I consider the use of sleep medications to be dangerous for these situations as it can lead to dependence and/or addiction, not to mention the hangover effects of the drugs.

The above situations exemplify loss of sleep as a symptom. But at what point does insomnia become a diagnosis rather than a symptom? Medical science does not address this issue. However, a carefully taken history will reveal the answer. The true insomniac has had sleep problems dating back to young adulthood and sometimes even earlier. Sleep remedies of many varieties have been tried such as medications, sleep hygiene, exercise, meditation, psychotherapy; and while all of these help for a while, the relief is short-lived. The individual still sleeps fitfully and sometimes not at all. There may be difficulty falling asleep or staying asleep or both.

I have noticed a curious discrepancy in this group of insomniacs. While all of them suffer through sleepless nights, about half seem to have good mood and energy during the waking hours and are productive in their work and private lives. They appear not to need much sleep in order to function well. The other half, alas, not only suffers throughout the night, but feels miserable during waking hours as well. Every chore is onerous. Fatigue and irritability, although sometimes kept hidden, are constant companions. It is almost as if these people are depressed, yet on the occasions when they do get a good night's sleep, they are highly functional and enjoy life. It may be that these individuals, unlike the other half, do need the recommended 7 or 8 hours sleep but just can't seem to get it.

Is there anything that can be done to 'cure' this variety of chronic insomnia? I am not an expert on sleep aids. This includes mechanical devices as well as tonics, lotions, potions, oils and herbs. I have never known anyone with severe insomnia who affected a cure with any of this. The search for such a cure has been a pet project of mine for several decades and I have to admit that I have not found the answer. However, I have identified a number of interventions that are of long term benefit to most insomnia sufferers, and I offer them to you along with my good wishes. Some of the suggestions can be life-altering (even if you don't wind up sleeping better), while others are little pearls of helpful wisdom accumulated from my own experience and that of many resourceful patients.

I will assume that you have already tried the usual 'sleep hygiene' advice widely available online and in print. If not, please do so, as it makes good sense. These measures by themselves do not induce sleep, but they are pre-requisites for anyone seeking relief from chronic or recurrent insomnia. Once you are in bed, turn your clock to the wall and do not look at it again until morning. In this way, you will avoid the 'ohmygod, I'm still not asleep' panic.

Nutritional:

If you feel hungry in the night, have a snack. I have found milk and honey or bananas and yogurt to be the most helpful and both are easily digested. This type of snack increases the availability of the amino acid tryptophan, which helps induce sleep. Otherwise it is a good idea to avoid eating within two hours of bedtime. Avoid eating heavy, fried or spicy foods and avoid drinking alcohol or caffeinated drinks in the evening.

Melatonin can be helpful; I have noticed that the research on melatonin shows that 'less is more.' That is, the most useful dosage is 0.3 mg at bedtime, rather than anything larger. In those studies, the low dose was the most effective at promoting sleep and produced minimal side effects. Valerian root is another sleep aid that works for some people. *Don't take either valerian or melatonin if you are taking a prescription sleep medication.*

Exercises:

Learn to become a more expressive person, so that feelings flow freely though your body. Try all the expressive exercises detailed in Chapter 47. If this does not work for you, seek the help of a body-oriented psychotherapist.

Learn a few lullabies and sing them out loud to yourself while in bed. Singing is a form of expression and also helps to interrupt the cycle of worry, anxiety and sleeplessness. This advice is very different from listening to soft music or relaxation tapes because it actively engages the non-thinking parts of your brain.

Try the sleep promoting breath exercise detailed in Chapter 45, Exercise 2.

If you have a spouse or mate who is willing, have him or her sit at the foot of your bed and hold your feet firmly in their hands for at least ten minutes. Do not talk.

No matter what exercise routines you normally practice, do the following in addition. An hour before bedtime, go outside and walk briskly for ten minutes.

This exercise, suggested by a friend, actually works for some hard-core insomniacs. Take a notebook and pen/pencil to bed. As you lie awake, force yourself to record every thought, image, feeling and sensation you experience. Keep this up and you may find yourself waking up a few hours later with the pencil still in your hand.

Going to the Source:

Practice meditation on a daily basis. You can use any of the methods listed in Chapter 50. You will find after a number of weeks of regular practice that even if your nights are still difficult, your days will be easier and more productive. If so, make this a life-long commitment as it will serve you well in all areas of your life. If you should happen to fall asleep during the meditation, you will awake feeling very refreshed.

If you are aware of having dreams from time to time, try to capture them and record them in a dream journal. Then, during your wakeful nights, try to re-create those dreams in your mind, with the intention of having more dreams with the same or similar content.

Other Interventions:

Lying awake in the dark of night when the rest of the world is asleep feels very lonely and it is true that misery loves company; so, if you know a fellow sufferer with whom you can commiserate, it is reassuring. Even if you can't talk to that person until the next day, it still helps to know you are not alone. Do not make the mistake of complaining to anyone who does not have the same problem – they do not understand and no matter how well-meaning, they trivialize your problem.

Try a few sessions of acupuncture. Be sure to tell the practitioner that your goal is to sleep better. If it does not work well and consistently after six sessions, it will probably not be useful to continue.

29 INTERCOURSE PAIN

For your physicians have expressly charged,
In peril to incur your former malady,
That I should yet absent me from your bed.
- Wm.Shakespeare, Taming of the Shrew

Also known as dyspareunia, painful intercourse is probably more common than is generally thought. We should not confuse this condition with lack of sexual desire in women, which can also lead to painful intercourse. If there is no desire, there will be little if any lubrication and opening, and this of course can predispose one to pain on penetration. Please see Chapter 27 - Impotence for remarks on lack of sexual desire in women and suggestions for treatment.

The most common 'medical' condition causing dyspareunia in women beyond middle age is hormonal imbalance, most likely low estrogen levels which in turn affect both desire for intercourse and the status of the vaginal tissues. Gynecologists can be of some help in this regard. But please also see Chapter 49 - Sexual

Exercises. Some of these exercises can be useful in stimulating desire and lubrication.

Young women who experience painful intercourse despite having a desire for sexual activity present the biggest challenge. In my opinion this condition almost always originates with tense pelvic musculature. *Medical conditions should be ruled out (e.g. infection, cysts, etc)*. The tense pelvis I am referring to here is a chronic, long-standing problem. It probably has a psychological origin, such as sexual abuse, shame, fear of punishment and so forth but I have not found talk therapy alone to be helpful in overcoming this type of tension and pain.

How do you know if you have a tight, constricted pelvis? If you are a young woman, you might have no symptoms from this problem other than painful intercourse. One sign that tension is present is an inability to imitate the pelvic movements of a belly-dancer. Try it and see. Another sign is your method of achieving orgasm through masturbation. If you find that the closer you get to orgasm, the more 'quiet' you become, in terms of sound and movement of the pelvis, you probably have a lot of pelvic tension. For some women, the only way they can get close to orgasm is by holding their pelvis thrust forward in a rigidly-maintained position. This is a sure sign that your pelvis is not free and open, and could well be the cause of your intercourse pain.

If there is a lot of tension in your pelvis, is there anything you can do about it yourself without getting help from a body-oriented therapist? Probably, but there are several 'pre-conditions.' The first is that you genuinely desire sexual intercourse. This is not the same as thinking you should want sex. It is a longing you can feel in your body. The second condition is that you truly believe that sex is not 'dirty' but is a normal, healthy part of being alive. Third, when you *imagine* opening up to penetration by a man's penis, you experience no fear.

There is no shame in not being able to meet these conditions. It is simply an indication that you will make better progress by seeking therapy prior to or along with any self-care interventions you wish to try.

Nutritional:

Regardless of the cause of your dyspareunia, eating well will support your healing and healthy sexuality. If you suffer from muscle spasms in the pelvic region, make sure that you are eating plenty of magnesium and zinc-rich foods (e.g. leafy greens, oysters, beans, seeds and nuts – especially walnuts), particularly if you are taking a calcium supplement. General inflammation can also cause pain. If you are still experiencing issues after a few weeks of following the 7 Guidelines for Eating Well in Chapter 3, it may be helpful to try the anti-inflammatory diet described in Chapter 52. You may also find it helpful to follow guidelines in the section on Depression, as these two problems can be related.

Some cases of dyspareunia are related to yeast or urinary tract infections (see Chapter 43 – Urinary Tract Infections). To eliminate yeast, cut sugar and starches out of your diet and drink cran-water (dilute unsweetened cranberry juice concentrate) for a week or two. Eating yogurt or fermented foods helps the body keep yeast under control. Staying well-hydrated can help with vaginal dryness, as can using a water-based lubricant. Hormone balance is also important, so I recommend staying away from soy, microwaved foods and food and drink in plastic containers, as these contain compounds which mimic hormones.

Exercises:

Try all of the sexual exercises in Chapter 49 to see which ones are most helpful to you.

Treat yourself to a whole body self-massage with warm sesame oil, daily.

Pelvic release work: Your pain may be caused by trigger points or adhesions – inflammation or scar tissue following trauma or surgery. Pelvic release work is a specific practice of body work aimed at releasing these trigger points and adhesions in the area of the pelvis, sexual organs and anus. For most people, this work also triggers the release of strong emotions. Successful pelvic release work can powerfully transform one's sexuality and have great benefit to other areas of life. The techniques of pelvic release can be taught by a skilled pelvic release practitioner. Try a self-care experiment to determine if this might be helpful for you.

Using your index finger, gently probe the area of your pelvis until you find a sore spot. Determine exactly where the worst pain appears and GENTLY hold your finger still on that spot. You may feel heat or pulsation under your finger. This is normal. Remember to breathe and allow any emotions to come. After one to two minutes, gently massage the spot and see if the pain is lessened. If so, you have just released a trigger point! You can repeat this self-care technique to find and release other trigger points. Ask a trusted intimate partner to help with areas in the vagina that are difficult to reach yourself. The key is to move slowly, touch gently, and give yourself time to experience emotions that may need to be expressed along with the release of the physical trigger point. Stop any individual session before you feel drained. You can always start again another time.

Full body relaxation: Lie on a comfortable but firm mat on the floor. Put a small pillow under your head or neck, whichever feels better. Begin by tensing the muscles of your feet and, while holding that, progressively tighten the muscles of your legs, pelvis, abdomen, chest, back, hands, arms and shoulders, neck, face and scalp. Keep breathing while holding the tension for as long as you can. Then release the tension slowly, starting with your feet, and let the relaxation spread upwards into the rest of your body.

When you have released all the tension in your body, feel the 'letting go' sensation and let it get deeper and deeper each time you exhale. Close your eyes and imagine that you are sinking into the mat, letting go more and more. Try to 'see' and feel the profound relaxation of all your muscles and joints. Maintain that restful posture for at least three minutes. When you get up off the floor, try to carry that relaxed feeling with you for a few moments.

Going to the Source:

First, do a ten minute meditation. Then, lie on a mat or a very firm bed and practice the full body relaxation technique described above. When your body is fully relaxed, allow yourself to have a sexual fantasy. Without judgment, imagine a scenario that turns you on. As you begin to become aroused, allow your breathing to become fuller, free and easy. Let yourself 'moan' with exhalation. At the same time, rock your pelvis very slightly forward and back. Let the movement be small, but free and easy, just like your breath. When you become really aroused, use your fingers to stimulate your 'erogenous' zones, usually mouth, nipples and clitoris. Keep the breath and pelvic rocking going while you do this. If you feel your pelvis becoming rigid, slowly bring the exercise to a stop and return to it another day. Do not give into the temptation to bring yourself to orgasm the 'old' way. Be patient with yourself and gradually you will find a way to 'open' to the experience, and soon to joyful, pain-free intercourse.

Note: if you find during the course of this exercise, that you are beginning to cry, please allow yourself full expression of that emotion. Do not cut it off or try to figure out why you are crying. A full-body sobbing can do more to release the tension than any of the exercises outlined here.

30 LEG CRAMPS AND RESTLESS LEGS

All the wild trash of sleep, without the rest.
- Edward Young

Leg Cramps

These are two separate disorders. Leg cramps occur primarily in older men and women, mostly at night. They are probably due to an imbalance in blood chemistry. In my experience the problem is unrelated to psychological issues or to exercise. The self-care approach is nutritional and is outlined below.

A word of caution: Do not confuse leg cramps, which occur mostly at night, with the severe cramping pain that occurs in some people while walking. This pain is called Intermittant Claudication, occurs primarily in the calf muscles, and is due to inadequate blood supply to those muscles. It requires expert medical attention.

Nutritional:

Leg cramps can often be solved by resting, drinking plenty of fluids and following the 7 Guidelines for Eating Well in Chapter 3. If leg cramps persist after a few weeks of this, then the next step is to make sure the balance of calcium, magnesium, potassium and sodium in the diet is correct. Stop eating and drinking things that demineralize your body. Sugar and sweets, alcohol, refined grains, MSG, aspartame, caffeine, and phosphoric acid in Coke and other soda bind calcium, magnesium, zinc and other minerals in the stomach and intestine. These minerals are then eliminated from the body.

If you are taking any prescriptions that promote calcium loss, have known hormonal diseases or imbalances, celiac disease or other intestinal conditions that interfere with calcium absorption, or have leg cramps or spasms primarily on the left side, then try increasing calcium-rich foods (e.g. leafy greens, dairy, sesame, nuts and seeds, molasses, papaya, etc.).

If your cramps are primarily on the right side and improve when you increase calcium, then try eating more foods rich in sodium (e.g. celery, pickles) or potassium (e.g. bananas) to find the proper balance. If right-sided leg cramps are not improved by increasing calcium, it generally indicates that you need more magnesium and you should eat more magnesium-rich foods. Random self-supplementation of the wrong vitamins and minerals can make things worse, so concentrate on food sources and give your body at least a week to adapt to each change. Keep a journal and note what you're eating, how you feel and how severe your leg cramps are each day.

A tea made from red raspberry leaf which contains vitamins, calcium, potassium, iron and fragrine (an alkaloid that nourishes muscles) can be helpful. Vitamin D-rich nettle leaf tea (traditionally used as an aid to kidney function) can ease pregnancy-related muscle spasms and leg cramps. Taurine (found in eggs, fish, meat, milk and sea vegetables) can be somewhat helpful for "sleep starts" if combined with a reduction in alcohol, caffeine, and white sugar.

Avoid eating:
- Alcohol and caffeine,
- Processed, fast and junk foods.
- Excessive sugar.

Eat more:
Foods rich in minerals Calcium, Magnesium, Phosphorus and Potassium, while increasing water consumption between meals.

Restless Legs

The symptom complex known as Restless Legs is another example of the medical profession creating a disease where none exists. There are no objective signs on physical exam and no abnormal laboratory tests to make the diagnosis. As with the other 'non-diseases,' prescription medication is usually dispensed, adding another unnecessary risk to the patient's well-being.

Restless legs occur mostly at night or other times when the person is trying to rest. The problem affects both sexes equally. *We are not referring here to the type of restless leg problem that occurs in pregnant women. In those cases you should consult your Ob/Gyn.* The problem can occur at any age. The word restless describes quite well the experience of the sufferer, who settles down for night's sleep only to find that his legs have a mind of their own. The legs seem to want to move, but moving them affords no relief from the irritable sensations. Getting out of bed and exercising helps somewhat, but is inconvenient and not all that reliable.

The problem can be seen as 'too much energy' in the legs. The situation is similar to a person who can't fall asleep because of constant mental activity, but the approach to symptom relief is much different. Self-care is all that is necessary if one is willing to take the time.

Nutritional:

Cleaning up your diet can help a great deal with restless legs. Follow the 7 Guidelines for Eating Well in Chapter 3, cut out caffeine and artificial sweeteners and cut back on alcohol and sugar. Iron deficiency is highly correlated, so eat iron-rich foods like red meat (which provides the most bio-available source of iron) along with foods rich in vitamin A (e.g. brightly colored fruits and vegetables) and folate (e.g. broccoli and leafy greens). Magnesium-rich foods can also help restless legs relax.

Exercises:

An hour before bedtime, perform the leg slamming exercise (Exercise 3b in Chapter 47) followed by the hanging over exercise (Exercise 1 in Chapter 46). These two exercises should dispel all or most of the excess energy in the legs and allow restful sleep.

If you prefer, there is another technique which is faster and can be done just before getting into bed. Most people seem unwilling to do it, however. It is a hydrotherapy method which results in bringing into balance the autonomic nervous system in the lower half of the body.

Obtain a medium size plastic tub, big enough and deep enough for you to sit in with your *legs outside the tub*. Place it on the floor of the shower and fill it with *very* cold water, about 6-8 inches deep. Sit in the tub (the water should reach just below your navel) for three minutes by the clock. Then dry off and go immediately to bed. This really works for restless legs and is also helpful for hemorrhoids and prostate enlargement.

31 MEMORY LOSS

Happiness is good health and a bad memory.
- Paul Newman

We all suffer memory loss to some degree as we get older. It is a normal part of aging and should not be confused with Alzheimer's disease which will not be dealt with in this book. Memory loss is troublesome in proportion to how we view ourselves. For some people, not being able to remember someone's name or where we left our glasses or being unable to recall who played the lead in a movie we saw last night is not a big deal. We laugh, call it a 'senior moment' and ask a friend for the information.

For others, those lapses represent a personal failure, a source of great distress. They ruminate about the problem, refuse to ask another person to jog their memory, and try to force themselves to recall the item in question. The harder they try, the more frustrated they become. This in turn results in anxiety, worsening the memory deficit.

I have found it to be useless to try to convince the latter group to relax and accept their faulty memory, to view it as a normal part of aging. They seek answers from the medical profession, which has nothing to offer in this instance.

Memory loss also seems to be associated with medications. I have observed that the more prescription drugs a person is taking, the more likely they are to have difficulties with cognition. This is especially true in older patients, who are the ones most likely to be ingesting multiple medications. While it is obvious that sleeping pills and tranquilizers are the worst offenders, I suspect that many other drugs are culpable. If you are following the guidelines in this book toward a more natural approach to healing, you may find that you will be able *(only upon the advice of your doctor)* to reduce the dose and/or number of your meds with a resulting increase in mental clarity and memory.

Whichever category of mis-rememberers you fall into, there is a lot you can do to ameliorate (though not cure) the problem. Prevention is the key here, so I would suggest that at the earliest sign that your mind is not as sharp as it used to be, begin the self-care program outlined below.

Nutritional:

In addition to aging, common causes of memory loss include poor nutrition, lack of sleep, depression, stress and anxiety, allergies, exposure to toxins and hormonal imbalances. Following the 7 Guidelines for Eating Well in Chapter 3 will improve things immediately. Overeating or eating processed, fast and junk foods will make matters worse. Keep sugar and sodium intake low and your memory will function much better.

Your body depends upon certain nutrients in your diet to function properly and that is certainly true of memory. Vitamins A and C help the body combat toxins and free radicals that damage brain cells. Omega 3 fatty acids, vitamins B and E and minerals selenium, iron and zinc are crucial for nerve and brain health, concentration and memory. The best sources of these nutrients are fruits and vegetables, liver, oysters and walnuts, fatty fish like salmon, mackerel, lake trout, herring, sardines, and albacore tuna, pastured meat and flaxseed. The choline in eggs helps the body make acetylcholine which is associated with slowing age-related memory loss. Garlic and ginkgo biloba increase blood flow to the brain, improving cognition and memory.

Include a high-protein food (eggs, meat, dairy, beans) with breakfast and a high-fiber source such as whole vegetables or fruit at every meal to improve memory and enhance attention throughout the day. While there is no research to show that drinking water improves our memory, it has been shown that even a small amount of dehydration leads to confusion and memory problems.

Excessive alcohol intake is toxic to brain cells, and illicit drugs such as marijuana, ecstasy, and cocaine block the function of neurotransmitters needed for memory. Toxins in the home and workplace can also cause memory loss or inability to concentrate including:

- lead in drinking water or paint in older homes,
- mercury in paints, dyes and inks,
- carbon monoxide leaking from home heaters,
- chemicals in pesticides and hobby materials.

Avoid eating:
- Alcohol and caffeine,
- Processed, fast and junk foods.
- Excessive sugar and salt.

Eat more:
- Fresh fruits and vegetables, walnuts,
- Pastured meat, liver and wild seafood,
- Breakfast, eggs.

Exercises:

In my opinion, most of the advice given in the popular press, for example in the AARP magazine, is sound. Tasks such as crossword puzzles, word and number games, adding columns of figures by 'hand,' all seem to be good ideas. Less TV and more reading also is helpful. There are a few less obvious techniques that I have found useful. They are based on stimulating other parts of the brain in addition to the usual left-brain exercises.

Singing: Copy the lyrics of a favorite song onto a sheet of paper. Then, stanza by stanza commit the words of the song to memory by singing it out loud. Do not try to recall the lines in your head. Keep singing the song out-loud until you remember it so well that you can sing it while doing something else – dishes, driving the car, etc.

Patterning Exercise: The first of these is the walking technique. It is the same as the walking meditation described in Chapter 50. Coordinating the voice and breath with rhythmic walking stimulates many areas of the brain. It is also very calming, once you have mastered the technique. Also very useful is the finger technique, which is also a form of meditation described in Chapter 48. It combines chanting, finger movements and leg movements all at once. These are both fun to do once you have learned them.

Paying attention: Giving your full attention to something or someone seems to be becoming a lost art. In the age of multi-tasking and device dependency, it is refreshing to find someone who seems to be giving you their full attention when you are interacting with them. When we are fully present for another person, it inspires trust and confidence. Clearly, it enhances the quality of any relationship, professional or personal. But in addition, it helps with our memory.

Let us use the example of being introduced to another person. If you want to remember that person's name and some relevant information about them, pay attention. How? First, stop whatever else you are doing; clear your mind of the previous activity. Next look directly at the person being introduced and listen carefully to his name. Repeat his or her name out loud and also 'see' it written out on the tablet of your mind. Then, talk less and listen (and see) more. People will love you for it and you will absorb and retain more.

32 NECK PAIN

*Appearances are deceptive. I knew a man who
acquired a reputation for dignity because he
had muscular rheumatism in the neck.*
- J. Chalmers Da Costa

Chronic or recurrent neck pain is very common.
While it does not result in as much acute disability as
low back pain, it certainly interferes with the quality of
life. In my opinion, the underlying cause is the same as
that for back pain: chronic muscular tension. While this
type of tension can be tolerated for years, causing
nothing more than a 'pain in the neck,' eventually it can
result in serious pathology requiring surgical
intervention. The reason for this is that the ongoing
tension in the muscles exerts pressure on the nerves
which exit the spinal cord through the vertebrae in our
neck, eventually causing damage to them. There are also
changes in the bony structure of the neck, resulting in
more compression on the same nerves. Sometimes the
problem is so severe that it can interfere with blood
flow through the arteries to the head.

There is very little your doctor can do for neck pain before it results in serious pathology. Pain medication is usually prescribed but this just masks the symptoms and does nothing to relieve the chronic tension.

People often seek help from a chiropractor for neck problems. The chiropractor tells you that the bones of your neck are 'out of alignment,' which may well be true (due to the pull of the tense muscles), and then 'cracks' your neck, sometimes resulting in temporary relief of the pain. But this process also does nothing to relieve the chronic tension.

Also, in my experience, massage therapy is not effective except as a transient pain and tension reliever. The therapist works to relieve the tension in the muscles and indeed may achieve a state of temporary relaxation of those muscles. However, if the underlying reasons for the neck tension are not addressed, the tension returns quickly and sometimes with increased intensity.

How then can we relieve the chronic tension safely and effectively? The answer lies in discovering for ourselves the source of the tension. A young man of my acquaintance suffers from recurrent bouts of severe neck pain. Over the years he has learned that when the neck pain recurs, it means that he has not effectively dealt with a stressful situation in his life. Usually one or two visits with his psychotherapist is all it takes to relieve the pain and get on with his life. We will deal with how to do this for yourself in the section on Going to the Source (see below). In the meantime, there are certain exercises that are somewhat helpful in letting go of the tension.

Nutritional:

None.

Exercises:

Practice the stand/bend exercise (Exercise 1, Chapter 46) every day, paying particular attention to letting the head hang freely.

The next exercise can be called the Big Shrug. In a sitting or standing position, tilt your head back on your shoulders while raising the shoulders up toward the ears. At the same time, jut your lower jaw forward, pushing it toward the ceiling, and reach up with your lips as though you were trying to kiss the sky. Hold this pose for ten seconds while continuing to breathe easily. Then very slowly reverse the process, relaxing the lips and jaw, and letting the shoulders down gradually. Let the head fall forward so that your chin rests on your chest. Appreciate the 'letting go' feeling. Now repeat the exercise two more times slowly, remembering to keep breathing.

A wonderful tension reliever for the neck requires the assistance of another person. Anyone whom you trust will do. Lie on your back on a high bed with your head near the foot of the bed. You can also use a massage table, which works even better. Your trusted partner sits at the foot of the bed and cradles your head in her/his hands. He or she gently raises your head just an inch or so off the mattress and continues to hold for about five minutes. This exercise will only work if you can totally give into the other person's support: *you must not help in any way.*

Another version of this which I like even better is this. Your assistant sits on the floor with her back against the wall. You lie on the floor between her legs with your head and shoulders resting against her chest. She then crosses her arms over your chest in a sort of reverse hug. Both of you fully 'let go' in your bodies and remain in this position for as long as possible, at a minimum five minutes. This exercise is the closest you can come (as an adult) to being taken care of by a good mother, letting the cares of the world fade away as you are held in her arms. If the exercise brings on tears, give into that as much as you can as that also enhances the release of tension.

Going to the Source:

As I have mentioned many times before, the regular practice of meditation will be helpful in relieving chronic tension anywhere in your body. However, please do not try to use meditation as medication. That is, don't expect it to give you lasting relief if you only do it when you are hurting. Meditation has all kinds of health benefits as well as promoting personal and spiritual growth, but only if it is a part of your daily routine for the rest of your life.

But you can use a meditative technique to help you get to the source of your chronic neck tension and pain. I have found that most often the neck tension results from trying to 'keep your head on straight.' In other words, you fear losing your head so you cling tightly to it with the muscles of your neck. Go inside and try to imagine how you would act if you 'lost your head.' Would you be 'crying your head off' or perhaps 'blowing your top' at someone.

These colloquial metaphors exist because they express essential truths. In the safety of your own private space, in a meditative posture, allow yourself to imagine expressing your rage or your grief or your longing. "See" yourself doing it. If this brings up a lot of feelings that frighten you, work for a while with a psychotherapist. Letting the feelings flow is NOT the same as acting them out. If you can find a way to let the feeling and energy flow through your body enough times, the tension and pain will fade away.

33 PREMATURE EJACULATION

Whenever it (semen) is emitted to excess, the
body becomes consumed, its strength
terminates, and its life perishes.
- Maimonides

Premature Ejaculation (PE) is included in this book because this problem is known to occur in about 30% of men. If one in three men suffer from this condition, should we be using words like problem, condition and suffer? In other words, is it simply normal for some men to ejaculate rapidly after penetration of a woman's vagina?

Although a diagnosis of PE is defined by most physicians and sex therapists as the inability to prolong intercourse for more than one minute after entry, recent research from evidenced based medicine indicates that rapid ejaculation is most likely a variation of normal, the lower end of the curve from quick to prolonged, and that the difficulties associated with it are largely a matter of male pride and female dissatisfaction.

Researchers tend to separate men with PE into two groups, primary and secondary. Men with secondary PE have had a so-called normal ejaculation pattern in the past and their current problem is thought to be 'secondary' to other issues in their life, most likely relationship problems, but sometimes health issues. For this group, the path to 'cure' is obvious: correct the underlying issue.

Men in the primary PE group have had the problem since puberty and it is unrelated to the type sexual relationship one has with one's partner. In the past, it was thought have a psychological basis, with theories ranging from Oedipal to peer pressure. None of these theories have been borne out by modern research methods. Psychotherapy is useful to deal with the humiliation these men sometimes feel, but is decidedly not helpful in prolonging intercourse time.

In fashion with the current trend in conventional medicine, PE has now been 'proven' to be due to neurobiological variability and related in a complex way to neurotransmitters. The proof will be in the pudding, the recipe for which should be to see if the recent studies stand up to independent replication. Alas, that is not likely to happen, as the current 'standard of care' is that primary PE should be treated with SSRI type pharmaceuticals; that is, anti-depressants. These probably do work, because as we noted in the chapter on impotence, libido is depressed by these medications. I would recommend their use with as much enthusiasm as I have expressed in their use for depression: if it works, and you can handle the side-effects, go for it. But please see the caveat in Chapter 3 about the use of multiple prescription medications.

Television, movies and the internet would have us believe that young men spend a great deal of time talking with each other about their sexual prowess. I don't see that happening in real life. I have never heard, in or out of the office, a guy complain that he 'comes too fast.' So I have had little experience in trying to be helpful in this situation. But I would like to offer a couple of observations that might prove helpful to some of you with primary PE who are eager for a solution. These suggestions are based on my knowledge of Bioenergetics and energetic flow through the body.

If you are someone who thinks about sex a lot, is easily aroused and very genitally focused, then when the time comes for penetration, you are already aroused almost to the point of orgasm. Practicing a bunch of techniques to delay ejaculation is not likely to work. What may help is if you can find a way make sex less important in your life. Do you find real pleasure and excitement in other activities? I'm talking about the kind of excitement that gets your energy flowing – eyes bright, skin flushed and feeling a bit high. If not, try to cultivate something in your life that fills that description. For some it might be music or dancing. What about tennis? I know some guys who get that way watching their favorite college basketball team. What about poker? See if you can get 'aroused' by something other than sex. If you can find that in your life, sex may become just another pleasurable activity for you, one in which you enjoy yourself without worrying about your performance.

Tantric sexology talks a great deal about methods of prolonging sexual pleasure and delaying orgasm based on learning to relax in states of high arousal. This can be done in the privacy of your own home by yourself or with a partner. Check yourself out next time you are aroused and observe whether the muscles around your belly, thighs, pelvis and buttocks are tight and tense. Is your pelvis thrust forward? When you masturbate, do you keep your pelvis in that pushed forward position and are the muscles of your perineum (between anus and penis) tightly held? If this is the case, take a deep breath, exhale slowly through your mouth and release all the tension in those areas. Let your pelvis 'hang' in the midline. Continue your masturbation without the associated tension. It may be somewhat less intensely pleasurable but you will probably go a lot longer before you come. If this works and you practice it often, you may find that it carries over into the bedroom with your partner.

A word about humiliation is in order here. It is easy to feel humiliated when you are 'spent' before your girlfriend is barely aroused. But if you really think about it, unless your partner is belittling you (in which case dump her right away), you can turn this around. Think of yourself as you really are, passionate and virile – certainly you are not impotent – and remember that your 'release time' is not an indication of your masculinity. If you can stay out of the embarrassment and shame, you will find wonderful ways of satisfying your girlfriend and she will love you for it.

34 PREMENSTRUAL SYNDROME (PMS)

No one who is not female can be in a position
to make accurate statements about women.
- Otto Weininger

In the developed nations, pregnancy, childbirth and menopause have become medicalized. That is, these situations fall under the purview of the medical profession. It is not just the complications of pregnancy and childbirth that now seem to require management by a physician, but the entire process as well. So it is not at all surprising that women expect their doctors to be able to do something about the normal variations in their psyche and soma that occur as a result of monthly hormonal swings.

When women seek help from medical professionals for the changeable moods and bodily discomforts associated with their periods, doctors comply by writing a prescription. This implies that the patient does indeed have something wrong with them that requires changing, and so a new disease is born, a new myth created.

Before you slam the book shut, please believe that I do know how much some of you suffer with the symptoms of PMS and that I do concur that you deserve relief. If you read on, you will see that there is much to offer in the way of relief, but not in the ways you have come to expect. There is no quick fix, because nothing is broken. Analogies to auto mechanics when it comes to health have always annoyed me, but I will carry this one a little further: I think we can offer you a smoother ride.

Why do some women suffer so much more than others around the time of their menses? Is it that their hormonal levels are so different from their peers and therefore require treatment? No, that is not the problem. Are they perhaps especially *sensitive* to the changes occurring in their bodies? That seems to be at least part of the problem.

If you suffer from PMS, is it not your experience that you are generally a sensitive person and that the manifestations of your sensitivity become stronger before your period? If this is true for you, it may be unrealistic to expect to remain on an even keel throughout the entire month. Is it really necessary to pathologize your variability? Whether you agree or not with what I have said, you still deserve relief from the symptoms that have come to be called PMS. Here are several self-care approaches to the situation.

Nutritional:
Although you should follow the 7 Guidelines for Eating Well in Chapter 3 throughout the month, it is particularly important during the second half of your

cycle. Eat less saturated fat and avoid alcohol and highly processed-high food during this time. To ease PMS symptoms such as nervous tension, irritability, and mood swings symptoms, eat foods rich in vitamins A, B, C, D, calcium, chromium, magnesium, zinc and selenium (e.g. green leafy vegetables, broccoli and cauliflower, carrots, fruits and other vegetables, walnuts, brazil nuts, sunflower seeds, molasses, pasture-raised meat and liver, oysters, shrimp and other seafood).

Eat 4-6 small meals per day, reduce sodium and eat more protein in the morning and more carbohydrates towards the end of the day. This will prevent water retention, bloating, breast tenderness, lethargy and cravings.

Low back pain, joint pain, nausea, vomiting and uterine cramps can be caused by inflammation, food intolerances (e.g. gluten or dairy) or delayed food allergies. Keep a food journal and try an elimination diet to determine what causes you problems.

Avoid eating:
- Alcohol and caffeine,
- Processed, fast and junk foods.
- Excessive protein, sugar and salt.

Eat more:
- Fresh fruits and vegetables,
- Pastured meat (especially turkey), liver and wild seafood,
- Foods rich in vitamins A, B, C, D, zinc, selenium, magnesium and calcium.

Exercise:

Since the symptoms vary so much from one person to the next, it is difficult to generalize. I suggest that you let your body be your guide. For example, if you tend to be exhausted, rest more. On the other hand, if somatic irritability is a prominent feature, do more vigorous exercise.

No matter what your symptom complex, I want you to try the pelvic exercises outlined in Chapter 49. My experience is that if the pelvis is free and 'open,' there are fewer symptoms of PMS.

Going to the Source:

If you practice meditation on a regular basis you will find that the emotional and physical variabilities of PMS are much easier to tolerate and you will be able to remain on a relatively even keel throughout the month.

If, during your meditation, a particular mood or physical symptom comes up strongly, try the following approach. Instead of trying to control the symptom and remain calm and relaxed, turn your full attention to it. If it is a headache that is plaguing you, sit quietly in the meditative posture and open yourself fully to the experience of the headache. Let it 'take you over,' while you simply observe what is happening. I think you will be surprised with the results.

If it is a particular mood, or emotion, that comes up for you, do the same thing. Open yourself to being flooded with that particular feeling. Do not try to escape from it or push it down. Let it wash over and through you. Stay with the sensations until they subside naturally.

Mark J. Sicherman, M.D.

35 PROSTATE ENLARGEMENT (BENIGN PROSTATIC HYPERTROPHY OR BPH)

As men draw near the common goal
Can anything be sadder
Than he, who, master of his soul,
Is servant to his bladder?
- Anonymous

It is known from autopsy studies that almost all men develop an enlarged prostate after a certain age. It is a normal condition of aging. Despite this, some men remain free of symptoms. Others develop obstruction to urinary flow which can become very severe, along with other symptoms such as urgency, dribbling and even incontinence. When the condition becomes severe, removal (resection) of the prostate is recommended. This usually results in marked relief of symptoms but there is a significant risk of damage to certain nerves, resulting in impotence. I urge all men to consider the following self-cure methods at the first sign of prostatic enlargement. You do not need to have a doctor confirm the diagnosis before trying these interventions, *but if they do not work, be sure to see your physician.*

Nutritional:

Medications available for treatment of BPH are often accompanied with undesirable side effects, while altering diet and lifestyle may reduce the occurrence and severity of this condition with no negative side effects. Excess weight correlates with prostate problems. Body fat produces hormones and chemicals that increase inflammation and can make prostate issues worse. Follow the 7 Guidelines for Eating Well in Chapter 3, concentrating on whole fresh unrefined and unprocessed, vegetables, whole grains, seeds, nuts, olive and coconut oils, and cold-water fish (salmon, tuna, sardines, halibut, and mackerel). Eating organic food helps reduce exposure to hormones, pesticides, and herbicides which can affect the prostate. Avoid refined sugar and flour, artificial sweeteners, dairy products, deep-fried foods, fast and junk foods, hydrogenated oils, alcohol (especially beer), and caffeine. The anti-inflammatory diet in Chapter 52 can also be helpful.

Drinking lots of water between meals helps the body flush out toxins. Herbal teas made with saw palmetto, pygeum bark or stinging nettles may also be helpful. Prostate problems are made worse by eating trigger foods, which vary from person to person. Keep a food journal and try an elimination diet to determine what causes you problems.

Long-term prostate health is improved by increasing the minerals zinc and selenium in the diet. The prostate needs more zinc to function properly than other soft tissues in the body. High levels of zinc help many prostate diseases and even inhibit prostate cancer from growing and spreading to other parts of the body. Zinc (from pumpkin seeds, oysters, red meats) and selenium (from Brazil nuts, sunflower seeds, cashews and fresh tuna) work together to protect prostate health. Mineral imbalances are unlikely if one eats a variety of whole foods rather than taking mineral supplements. Vitamins A, B, C, E and magnesium are also important for prostate health so include lots of leafy greens and fresh fruit. Drinking alcohol reduces the body's store of zinc and vitamin B6. Beer in particular contains oestrogens which are high in men with BPH and block zinc from being absorbed by the intestines.

Avoid eating:
- Alcohol (especially beer) and caffeine,
- Processed, fast and junk foods.
- Excessive sugar and salt.

Eat more:
- Fresh fruits and vegetables,
- Pastured meat, liver and wild seafood,
- Foods rich in B vitamins along with C, A, D, zinc and selenium.

Exercises:
There is one technique that has worked so well for me and for several patients I have treated, that I urge you to try it despite your reservations. That is the cold Sitz bath. Please see the description in the section on Hemorrhoids in Chapter 23 – Gastrointestinal Problems. Follow the same process except sit longer in the cold water and repeat the technique as necessary during the daytime as well.

Going to the Source: none

A word about prostate cancer:

Perhaps it is medical heresy, but I have serious reservations about the benefits of the widely used PSA screening test for prostate cancer. When the test reveals elevated levels of PSA, multiple biopsies of the prostate gland are recommended for all men. To what end? Well, of course to detect prostate cancer in its earliest stages and then to remove or irradiate the offending organ. Certainly, this protocol should and apparently does reduce the mortality rate from prostate cancer. The more people you diagnose with early stage cancer, the more you save.

BUT, do we know what would have happened to those men with early stage prostate cancer if they did not get treated with this 'standard of care?' We do know that men over 65 are likely to die from some other disease before their prostate cancer does them in. In other words, in that age group, the protocol does not improve survival rates or reduce mortality rates. And the men who elect to do nothing do not run the considerable risk of impotence and incontinence which accompanies prostatectomy.

What about younger men? I do not have any answers, but I do have some observations. There seems to be a growing risk (or perhaps it is now more widely reported) of blood stream infection (septicemia) with the E.coli bacteria following multiple prostate biopsies. This infection can easily kill you, even if properly and promptly diagnosed and treated.

Then of course there is concern about the risks of removing the prostate in a relatively young man. I had one patient whose surgeon never even mentioned the possibility of impotence. This man was devastated by his loss of sexual competence. He became deeply depressed and reclusive.

It's possible that early detection is finding a lot of cancer that wouldn't need treatment or cause any problems if left undetected. I offer these thoughts in hopes that some men, and hopefully some physicians, will take the risk of thinking outside the box, before following the 'standard of care' in all cases. Is it so heretical to take your individual priorities into account, to look at all the information and options, and to make a decision based on your individual circumstances? Don't let yourself be panicked to "get the cancer out" and deny yourself the time (and study) necessary to make a considered decision.

36 RAYNAUD'S DISEASE (AKA RAYNAUD'S PHENOMENON)

The veins unfilled, our blood is cold.
- Coriolanus

This condition occurs most often in women. Although it is sometimes associated with other 'autoimmune' disorders such as Rheumatoid Arthritis, the symptoms can occur as an isolated phenomenon. Constriction of the blood vessels to the periphery (hands and feet, sometimes the nose or ears) results on exposure to cold temperatures. The fingers turn white, then after a while, blue. When the blood supply opens up, and the fingertips are suffused with blood, a bright red color ensues. All stages of the process can be quite uncomfortable and if the condition is severe and prolonged, complications can occur.

It is also known that the blood vessel constriction can occur due to emotional upset, even when the ambient temperature is warm. This certainly supports the theory that the underlying problem is one of autonomic nervous system imbalance, in this case an 'over-reaction' of the sympathetic branch of this system, which typically results in a diminished blood supply to the periphery of the body.

Besides the potentially dangerous prescription medications that can be used to prevent or ameliorate the condition, much help can be gotten from a self-care approach designed to bring the autonomic nervous system into balance. Although not strictly in the category of self-care, I would also strongly recommend acupuncture on a regular basis as a preventive measure.

Nutritional:

Raynaud's symptoms can be significantly improved by following the 7 Guidelines for Eating Well in Chapter 3, getting regular exercise and avoiding triggers. Smoking, drinking alcohol and caffeine make Raynaud's worse in most people so avoid these.

The best nutrients for Raynaud's, omega-3 fatty acids, are found in abundance in seeds (especially flaxseed), nuts and wild cold-water fish. Niacin (vitamin B3) also improves blood flow and is high in green vegetables, seeds, mushrooms, seafood, meat, eggs, and dairy. Try cooking with warming spices like turmeric, cinnamon, cumin, cayenne, ginger, mustard, horseradish and garlic. Imagine wrapping your fingers around a warm cup of vegetable broth made by boiling your favorite chopped vegetables with fresh grated ginger, chopped garlic and a pinch of cayenne. For immediate relief you can even massage a paste of warm water, fresh ground mustard, ginger and cayenne into the skin during attacks.

Some people with Raynaud's may need to increase foods containing vitamin E or magnesium (e.g. green leafy vegetables, nuts or nut oils, dark chocolate) and for some the herb ginkgo biloba helps increase blood flow to the extremities. It's also a good idea to note which foods, drugs and situations trigger an attack by keeping a journal. For example, many people find that taking cold and flu remedies containing pseudoephedrine can bring on an attack of Raynaud's.

Avoid eating:
- Alcohol and caffeine,
- Trigger foods.

Eat more:
- Seeds (especially flaxseed), nuts and wild cold-water fish
- Green vegetables, warming spices,
- Foods rich in niacin, magnesium, vitamin E.

Exercises:
Here is a variation of a tai chi exercise that I would urge you to try. Stand with your feet eight inches apart, your knees slightly bent, and your weight slightly forward on the balls of the feet (do not lift the heels from the ground). Keep your spine straight and your head level. Bring your arms forward, keeping the elbows bent and fairly close to your body, until the fingertips of each hand approach the other hand, stopping when they are about three inches apart. It is as if you were holding a large beach ball at waist level.

Relax everything, 'hang loose.' Be conscious of letting go of tension in your jaw, neck, shoulders, arms, hands and belly. Breathe freely and easily as you stand. Try to maintain the position for at least five minutes. Do this every day. After a few days try to increase your time by one or two minutes until you can work up to fifteen minutes. While you are doing this exercise, keep your attention fully on the sensations in your body. DO NOT watch TV or carry on a conversation. If you do this regularly, you should notice an improvement in the Raynaud's symptoms within a week or two.

Also useful is this Hydrotherapy exercise, which may give you prompt relief. If performed daily, it brings the autonomic nervous system in the upper body into balance and should prevent further attacks. Follow this procedure at the end of your morning shower (please do not use this technique in the evening as it may be too stimulating and interfere with getting to sleep). Concentrate the stream of water by adjusting the shower head. Run the stream of hot water (as hot as you can comfortably tolerate) on the middle of your back, between your shoulder blades, for three minutes. Then turn the water temperature to very cold and spray the same area for one full minute. Next, return to hot and do another three minutes, followed by another full minute of cold. Always end with cold. If you are brave enough to do this on a daily basis, you should notice an improvement in your symptoms rather quickly and the relief should last the rest of the day. I have done this technique myself many times to relieve a tendency toward mild depression and it works well. The only way I can tolerate the cold spray is with a lot of hooting and hollering.

Going to the Source:
If you have good visualization skills, this technique should work very well for you. Sit in a meditative posture to elicit the relaxation response or until you feel a letting go in your body. Keep your hands open in

your lap, palms up or down. 'See' yourself breathing in warm golden sunlight through the top of your head and into your chest. Now slowly release the breath. 'See' and feel that golden warmth traveling down your arms and into your hands, suffusing them with a comfortable, warm sensation. Do this for at least ten breaths, until the fingers have regained normal color and temperature. This is also a good preventive technique.

37 SINUSITIS

The doctor of the future will give no
medication, but will interest his patients in the
care of the human frame, diet and in the cause
and prevention of disease.
- Thomas Edison

I did not include sinusitis under allergies because it deserves special consideration. Further, although more common in people with hay fever, sinus congestion and infection also occurs in the absence of allergies. It can complicate a 'cold,' prolonging the upper respiratory symptoms (post-nasal drip, cough, low-grade fever, malaise) for weeks.

The conventional treatment of sinusitis involves medications to dry up the mucous and antibiotics to resolve the infection. Unfortunately, there is no easy way for a physician to distinguish between congestion of the sinus cavities without infection from those cases with bacterial infection. Thus, antibiotics are used much more often than is necessary, resulting in gastrointestinal problems, yeast infestation and resistant strains of bacteria in many individuals.

Everyone gets a cold or other viral upper respiratory illness now and then. Our sinus cavities are congested during the course of such an illness, but they clear up as the other symptoms of the illness subside. Some of us however go on to develop chronic congestion of the sinuses and/or secondary bacterial infection of those cavities. Why? Because the sinuses do not drain the way they are supposed to. The connections between them and the nasal passages are blocked.

It has become evident to me that this blockage, this failure to drain properly, happens because of chronic tension in the muscles of the face, especially the para-nasal muscles between the cheekbone and the nose. I can offer no scientific proof of this statement, but sinus problems improve markedly in those individuals who have been taught to release the tension in those muscles.

If you suffer from chronic or recurrent sinus problems and are under conventional care for this condition, please ask your doctor not to prescribe antibiotics as the first line of defense. Also ask him or her if you might need an anti-fungal agent to deal with possible yeast (Candida) overgrowth in your sinuses and elsewhere in your body. I would also suggest that you consider acupuncture, which has a pretty good track record in dealing with chronic sinus problems.

Nutritional:
Follow the 7 Guidelines for Eating Well in Chapter 3 to improve general nutrition and health. If you also eliminate bread, beer, wine and any other fermented products along with all sources of sugar for 21 days,

you will greatly aid your body in eliminating any yeast over growth in your sinuses or elsewhere.

Exercises:

To find out if you have tense facial muscles that may be blocking your sinus drainage, perform the following experiment. Sitting straight in a chair, press the tips of your forefingers deep into the fleshy areas between the sides of your nose and your cheekbones. If you experience pain in addition to the sensation of pressure, then these muscles are tense. To release the tension, use the tips of your fingers to massage the area. Start at the top, just below the eyes, and run your fingers firmly down the sides of your nose, moving gradually outward toward the cheeks. The motion should be slowly down and out, and repeated at least ten times. Do this several times a day, even when you are not suffering from sinus congestion. You will know if you have been successful in releasing the tension when you no longer experience pain with pressure on the area.

Going to the Source:

Take some time to sit quietly and consider why your facial muscles might be tense. Are you smiling too much; that is, are you smiling when you don't really mean it. Has your smile become fixed in all social or professional engagements? Also, are you holding back tears? If you were to let go of all the tension in your face, would you feel sad and start to cry? If so, then that is exactly what you need to do, in the privacy and safety of your own space.

You can also use a visualization exercise to help open the sinuses. First, sit in a meditative posture for at least five minutes to elicit the relaxation response.

Then, with eyes closed, 'see' your sinuses being flooded with crystal clear water, draining away all the congestion and infection. Do this for one or two minutes and then 'see' golden rays of sunshine healing the insides of your sinuses, resulting in clear, healthy pink membranes.

38 SORE THROAT

He prayeth best who loveth best
All things both great and small.
The Streptococcus is the test –
I love it least of all.
- Wallace Wilson

Sore throat is one of most common presenting conditions in a doctor's office, especially with physicians who treat children. It occurs so frequently that it merits an extensive discussion here.

Parents seem especially worried about 'strep throat' in their kids and are eager to get antibiotic treatment as early as possible. There is only one way to make a definitive diagnosis of 'streptococcal pharyngitis' and that is with a throat culture. Most clinicians (myself included) feel that they can diagnose the condition by the appearance of the throat, the sound of the voice and the smell of the breath. If the child has fever, swollen glands in the neck and a stomach ache along with the other signs, we feel certain. However, studies show that we are wrong almost as often as we are right, and that we uselessly prescribe antibiotics in many cases.

Most of you are aware that the excessive use of antibiotics is detrimental to the patient and to the community at large. Development of resistant strains of bacteria, yeast infestation in the patient, and gastrointestinal disorders are some of the problems. I would urge you not to 'jump the gun' when it comes to your child's sore throat, or for that matter, your own.

If there is an inability to swallow liquids or to keep them down, if the fever is very high and persistent, if a red rash is present on the body, or if the patient is too sick to get out of bed, then there is cause for concern and the doctor should be consulted right away.

Otherwise, it is safe to wait three to five days to see which direction the illness is taking. If the fever and other symptoms are subsiding in that time frame, it is probably not strep throat or if it is, the body's defenses are handling it well. If symptoms persist beyond five days, certainly a visit to the doctor is warranted.

When a child or an adult experiences recurrent sore throats and/or very frequent respiratory infections of any sort, one should consider that the immune system may not be functioning optimally. There are certain tests your doctor can order to see if this is the case. Fortunately, most of the time these tests reveal nothing abnormal, but we are left wondering why the person is getting sick so often.

It has been my observation over many decades that there are reasons that underlie this problem that most practitioners do not consider. One reason that is easy to 'diagnose' and simple to treat is excessively dry air in the home (or workplace). If the humidity level is below 30%, the mucous membranes of the nose and throat tend to dry out, become irritated and therefore subject to infection. To correct the problem, obtain a high quality humidifier and keep the level in your home above 40%. You should notice less cough and scratchy throats within a couple of days.

Another more nebulous problem is allergies. In my opinion, undiagnosed food allergy is the culprit in many cases of recurrent upper respiratory infections. Food allergies not only wreak havoc on the immune system (this would not necessarily show up in standard tests of immune function) but also may cause an absorption problem, preventing the patient from getting enough essential nutrients to maintain good health. A certified nutritionist can be very helpful if you suspect that you or your child might have this problem.

Lastly, but probably most commonly, are the physiologic effects of stress. Stress has been clearly demonstrated to be detrimental to immune functioning. If immune function is compromised, we are more susceptible to infection. We do not have space here to attempt a full discussion of the effects of stress on the body, but it is important to note that stress can be physical, mental-emotional, and even spiritual. As we discussed in Chapter 5, if the stress cannot be avoided, there is a specific antidote to its ill-effects – meditation.

Nutritional:
Follow the 7 Guidelines for Eating Well in Chapter 3.

Exercise:
I believe that if you keep the voice flowing 'free and clear,' you will be less likely to experience sore throat and infection of the throat. Choose any of the voice

exercises in Chapter 45 and work towards opening up that part of your body.

Going to the Source:

As noted above, meditation is an antidote to the effects of stress on your body. The regular practice of a meditation technique should be helpful in preventing recurrent sore throats.

In children under 12, meditation is probably not appropriate. If kids at this tender age are experiencing too much stress in their lives, it is up to the parents to make the necessary changes in their children's lives so they get plenty of physical activity, enough sleep, and time to day-dream and play.

39 STUTTERING AND TICS

Whirled in a vortex that shall bring
The world to that destructive fire
Which burns before the ice-cap reigns.
That was a way of putting it—not very
satisfactory:
A periphrastic study in a worn-out poetical
fashion,
Leaving one still with the intolerable wrestle
With words and meanings.
- T.S. Eliot

We will confine our discussion of stuttering and tics to those occurring in childhood. This is when most of these problems have their onset and if they can be effectively dealt with early on, the person is less likely to experience the problem as an adult.

Many children go through a period when their desire to communicate outpaces their ability to put their thoughts into words. This results in an urgency which parents often mis-label as stuttering. It seems to occur most commonly in bright, energetic children during the pre-school years. A typical example is the little boy who tugs at his mother's sleeve, saying, "Mommy, I, I, I, I, I have to go potty." The child knows what he wants and knows the words for it, but his mind is so busy with other, more important things, that he can't be bothered to take the time to focus on what he's saying. Also, not unreasonably, he expects his mother to know what his needs are without his needing to ask. Often, the repeated word is 'why' or 'but.' This is sometimes referred to as "stammering."

This pattern is *not the same as stuttering*, which is an inability to form the word, resulting in a repetition of the first letter, or mouth movement with no sound at all. Along with this the child appears in distress and frustrated at not being able to communicate. True stuttering often has a neurological and/or psychological basis and should be evaluated by specialists in child development, child psychology, neurology and speech therapy.

The much more common condition called stammering requires only patience and reassurance on the part of the parent. If possible, the parent should find a way to calm themselves and the child for a moment, make eye contact and say, "Now, what did you want to tell Mommie?" In any case, the important thing is for the parent not to over-react, become anxious and communicate their tension to the child. The parent may want to discuss the 'problem' with an experienced pediatrician in order to be reassured that the child will outgrow the problem by first grade. Hopefully, the doctor will not over-react by sending the child for 'further testing and evaluation' by specialists.

The same reassurance is needed for parents of children who develop tics at sometime during childhood, most often in the middle years. I have no patience with physicians who tell these parents that their child's tic may be an early sign of Tourette's Syndrome, conjuring up for the poor mother images of their child as an adult, walking down the street cursing, grimacing and spitting.

It has been my experience that tics occur more frequently in children who are anxious. Therefore, the attention of the parent and the professional should be focused on the origins of the child's anxiety and on ways to reduce or eliminate it.

When a child develops a tic, it is important for the parent, and a professional if need be, to distinguish the tic, an involuntary activity, from repetitive, obsessive behaviors which are under voluntary control and which represent potentially serious emotional problems in the child. The latter group requires professional evaluation.

The typical 'tic' in childhood is a facial twitch or grimace around the eyes or mouth. The tic is intermittent and the child appears not to notice it, going about their business as if nothing is happening. It can also involve movements of the hands or fingers, and it is here where the distinction between a transient tic and compulsive behaviours may be difficult to determine. No harm will be done by a period of watchful waiting, during which every attempt should be made to reduce the stress level in the child's life. After a period of months, if the problem is still present, professional help should be sought.

40 TEMPOROMANDIBULAR JOINT DISORDER (TMJ)

The fathers have eaten sour grapes, and the
children's teeth are set on edge.
- Ezekiel 18:2

This diagnosis is often made by dentists or ENT specialists because patients complain of head, face and ear pain on the affected side. Chewing may be difficult and there is limited ability to open the mouth wide. It is thought to be due to overuse and/or spasm of the 'chewing' muscles resulting in damage to the TM joint. Most often it is blamed on chronic grinding of the teeth while sleeping. Various devices are prescribed to prevent nighttime teeth grinding and advice is given to rest the jaw muscles. Prescriptions are given for pain relievers, muscle relaxants and anti-inflammatory agents.

In my experience, the conventional approach is minimally effective in relieving symptoms and does nothing to deal with the underlying cause of TMJ. The condition is clearly due to chronic tension in the jaw muscles. While some physicians and dentists agree that 'stress' may underlie the muscular tension, their approach to that is pharmaceutical.

I have seen many patients with this condition, although they usually mention it in passing when consulting me for psychological or chronic physical problems. If I press my fingers firmly into the edge of the chewing muscles with the mouth slightly open, this causes excruciating pain to the patient. It also brings up a flash of anger which is obvious in their eyes and voice. It is this anger which is at the root of the problem.

Usually, persons suffering with this condition are *not* overtly angry people. In fact, they are often very 'smiley' and agreeable. They have learned since childhood to keep their mouth shut and put on a pleasant face. They have learned it so well that they are no longer hiding their anger; rather, they are totally unaware of it. However, they are acutely aware of their symptoms and are eager for relief.

If you suffer from symptoms of TMJ and wish to obtain relief, the techniques outlined below will relax the chronic tension in your jaw muscles. You do not have to deal with the underlying issues which brought on the problem, although if you are open to it, consultation with a body-centered psychotherapist can be very helpful and can help you avoid recurrences.

Exercises:

a. Use the anger releasing voice exercise (Exercise 3d in Chapter 47) and practice it every day for several weeks.

b. Open your mouth half way and grab your chin firmly between your thumb and forefinger. Keeping your mouth in the half open position, pull down hard with your hand as if trying to force your mouth open while at the same time use the jaw muscles to try to force the mouth closed. Maintain the pressure in both directions while exhaling forcefully. Make a sound like a lion's roar as you exhale. Keep this up for a minute or so, then gradually release the pressure. Do this one more time and when finished, gently massage the jaw muscles on the sides of your face.

This exercise, done regularly, is more effective than the devices prescribed by dentists for the problem. In addition to relaxing the muscles around the TMJ joint, the 'lion's roar' also provides a release of the pent-up anger and fear which contributes to jaw tension.

c. Sit with your jaw slightly open and massage your jaw muscles with the tips of your fingers. Do both sides of your face simultaneously, even if only one side is painful. Convey gentleness and caring to those muscles. Massage for about three minutes, three times a day.

d. If your pain is not yet so severe that it prevents you from chewing solid foods, the following exercise can have remarkably good results. Wash and peel a medium size carrot. Take a good sized bite of the carrot and *chew it very slowly and very deliberately until it is completely pulverized* before swallowing. Eat the whole carrot like this. This exercise is particularly helpful at releasing the chronically held-back anger that underlies TMJ.

Going to the Source:

If you are willing to learn and practice meditation, you will find it to be very helpful in the long run for this and many other symptoms. Select a method from Chapter 50 and practice every day.

The following technique is specific for TMJ problems. Sit in a meditative posture, close your eyes and let your jaw drop. Breathe freely and easily through your mouth. If possible let a slightly audible moan escape with each out breath. Don't worry if you drool a bit. Imagine yourself as someone who cares not at all about what others think of them. Maintain this posture for at least five minutes. Practice it whenever you have the chance.

41 TINNITUS

In my ears has been ringing and droning all
day,
Without ever a stop or a change.
- Thomas Hood, All in the Downs

Ringing in both ears is almost always a benign condition. It is however a very annoying problem which deserves attention because it interferes with conversation, concentration and sometimes even with sleep.

If you have persistent ringing in just one ear, it may indicate a more serious problem and should be evaluated by a physician. Also, if it is associated with a hearing loss, see an ENT physician or an audiologist.

Tinnitus occurs most commonly as a side effect of medications, prescription and over-the-counter. It is a well-known side effect of aspirin, even when taken in recommended dosage, but almost any drug seems capable of causing the problem.

If you are taking a drug for a short period of time and that drug is useful to you, you can ignore the tinnitus and be reassured that it will subside when you stop the medication. If, however, you are taking a drug indefinitely, you may want to determine if it is the cause of the ringing in your ears.

If it is a non-prescription drug, such as a non-steroidal anti-inflammatory agent, you can simply lower the dose or eliminate it altogether for several days to see if it was the cause of your tinnitus. If it is a prescription medication, check with your doctor to determine if it is safe to lower your dose. If you discover that in fact your medicine is the cause, ask your doctor to suggest an alternative.

Tinnitus is also sometimes associated with TMJ (see Chapter 40). In this instance, follow the suggestions for that condition to get relief. Even if you have not been diagnosed with TMJ, some of the exercises listed there may be helpful to you.

42 UPPER RESPIRATORY ILLNESS (URI) / COLDS

If you think that you have caught a cold, call
in a good doctor. Call in three good doctors
and play bridge.
- Robert Benchley

When I was a young doctor, I enjoyed telling patients, "the common cold, if left untreated, lasts seven days; with treatment, it lasts a week." While it is still true that there is no cure for the common cold, I am no longer able to reassure patients that it will last no longer than a week. We are now seeing so-called 'viral URI's' that are more severe in intensity and duration. Sometimes the symptoms come and go with a whimsy that defies explanation. And there seems to be an increase in the frequency of complications of the common cold, such as sinusitis and bronchitis.

One is tempted to blame this trend on new viruses or more virulent strains of the old viruses, but I suspect this is only part of the problem. My guess is that our millennial life-style has made the host (our bodies) more welcoming to the invaders. Our collective resistance has been lowered by the way we choose to live. And once we are infected, we have less healing resources to bring to bear against the virus.

There is a plethora of over-the-counter medications designed to bring relief to sufferers of the common cold, to control mucous production and reduce malaise (generalized aches and pains and fatigue). New medications always seem to work better than the old ones, but that is clearly the 'placebo effect.' If you think it is going to help, it will, at least for awhile. Be careful, there is no magic, and some of the drugs have potentially serious side effects. Even the alternative remedies – herbal, homeopathic or heavy metal suspensions – need to be used with caution. I would be especially cautious about putting anything in your nose except saline nose drops. Anything else could cause permanent damage to your sense of smell.

If you have only one or two colds per year, short-lived and without complications, consider yourself lucky. But for those of you with more frequent URI's and a tendency to complications, please consider the following self-care interventions.

Nutritional:

Obviously the better your immune system is functioning, the less likely you are to come down with a cold. Following the 7 Guidelines for Eating Well in Chapter 3 will prepare your immune system for cold season and should reduce both the severity and frequency. Be particularly mindful of reducing sugar and nightshade vegetable intake.

Once you've got a cold, there are several things you can do to lessen the suffering and get back to normal quicker. To relieve head and chest congestion and chills, a powerful warming anti-viral tea made from fresh-grated ginger and cayenne pepper mixed with two tablespoons of fresh lemon juice, a dash of honey and one or two gloves of fresh crushed garlic can provide relief. I'm also a believer in the power of chicken soup – if it is homemade and especially if it is made with love. As corny as this may sound, feeling loved can definitely improve immune function. Other than this, drink plenty of water, stay warm and rest.

Avoid eating:

- Sugar, junk food, fast food, sodas, alcohol, smoking,
- Nightshade vegetables (potatoes, tomatoes, eggplant) as these can suppress immune function in some people.

Eat more:

- Anti-virals such as garlic, onions, and homemade chicken soup,
- Warming spices such as ginger, cayenne, and turmeric,
- Vitamin-C rich foods such as green leafy vegetables, cabbage, cauliflower, broccoli, peppers, citrus fruits, and berries,
- Foods rich in omega-3 fatty acids, especially flaxseeds and cold water fish such as salmon and mackerel which can help ease nasal congestion and reduce inflammation.
- Whole foods rich in Vitamins A, C, E and minerals zinc and selenium which are

antioxidants that can help your immune system function properly.

Exercises:

Whatever your exercise routines are, please do less, or perhaps none at all, while you are suffering with a cold. You need rest and I do not believe, as some do, that you can 'bully' the virus out of your system. In fact, your attempt to do so may invite the virus to settle into other parts of your body and plague you for long periods. This is clearly not a science-based piece of advice, but I have seen it happen.

Going to the Source:

The cold virus or viruses seem to have an interesting and unusual relationship to 'stress.' The following scenario is typical. You are exposed to someone with a bad cold – they sneeze on your groceries or pump your hand in a hearty greeting. You are in the middle of a stressful week of appointments, meetings, commitments. You forget that you were 'contaminated' with the virus and feel just fine. When your stressful week is over, you put your feet up to relax for a few hours or a weekend, and wham, you are hit with a miserable cold. Cold viruses appear not to like acute stress, but beware if you are in a chronic stressful situation, a job you hate, going through a contentious divorce, etc. During this time you may experience one cold after another.

While meditation will do nothing at all for the common cold once you have acquired one, it can help boost your immune system during times of chronic stress. You will find that if you practice meditation on a very regular basis, you will experience fewer bouts of

upper respiratory illness and when they do occur, you
will heal faster.

43 URINARY TRACT INFECTIONS

Never accept a drink from a Urologist.
- Erma Bombeck

This condition is very common in women, but infrequent in men. In men, it is usually the urethra and prostate which become infected while in women it is most often the bladder. Once the urinary tract has become infected, there is little choice but to take antibiotics to clear the infection and to prevent it from ascending to the kidneys. A kidney infection, which is also called pyelonephritis, can be very severe and can cause lasting damage to this vital organ.

Early in the course of a urinary tract infection, if the symptoms are still mild, it is worth trying a nutritional remedy (see below) in hopes of avoiding the hazards of prescription antibiotics. But if there is no improvement in a couple of days, please contact your physician. On the other hand, if you are interested in *preventing* a UTI, the following self-care measures have a lot to offer.

Nutritional:

Following the 7 Guidelines for Eating Well in Chapter 3 will improve your general health and immune function, which will do much to help you prevent or resolve infections. It is fairly common knowledge that cranberry juice decreases the incidence of UTI and recent clinical studies confirm its preventative benefit in those with frequent infections. The best way to take cranberry is to purchase 100% cranberry juice (preferably organic) and mix it with plenty of water, adding liquid stevia to taste. This avoids the heavy dose of sugar included in commercial cranberry juice "cocktails." Drink several glasses of weak cran-water daily to clear a mild UTI, and one or two a day as a preventative. Add two teaspoons of unfiltered organic apple cider vinegar to an eight-ounce glass of cran-water for a powerful UTI-healing tonic.

Avoid junk foods, fast foods, commercial baked goods or sweets, sweetened fruit juices, sodas and other sweetened drinks. Also avoid coffee, alcohol and tobacco and cut down on possible allergens like wheat (gluten), dairy, and grains. Any of these can depress your immune function and make you more prone to infection. One exception to this is yogurt. The live cultures in yogurt help protect the body from infection. If you feel you might not be getting enough vitamin C, add more green leafy vegetables, citrus fruit and berries to your diet.

Avoid eating:
- Junk foods, fast foods, commercial baked goods or sweets.
- Sweetened fruit juices, sodas and other sweetened drinks, coffee, alcohol and tobacco.

- Food allergens like wheat (gluten), dairy, and grains.

Eat more:
- Cran-water from 100% organic cranberry concentrate, apple cider vinegar,
- Yogurt with live cultures,
- Green leafy vegetables, citrus fruits and berries.

Exercise:
If you are prone to UTI's and have been told that your infection is due to the bacteria E.Coli (the most common offender) and if your infections seem to follow sexual intercourse (also very common), then meticulous genital/perineal hygiene is indicated. Taking a shower before sex may seem like a turn-off, a destroyer of spontaneity. But consider that in both Tantric and Taoist traditions, careful washing and the use of essential oils prior to intimate contact heightens sensuality and enhances sexual pleasure.

There is another important consideration, especially for women, which is rarely talked about. If you are not really 'ready, willing and eager' for sex, don't do it. Genuine arousal results in the release of natural lubricants, which I believe are protective, directly or indirectly, against infection. It is clear that without lubrication, irritation of the mucosal tissues occurs, setting the stage for infection.

If lack of arousal is a chronic problem for you, please see the advice in the Chapter 27 - Impotence.

44 SELF CARE FOR CANCER ?!!!?

"Cancer is the emperor of all maladies, the king of our terrors."
- Siddhartha Mukerjee quoting a 19th century physician
More people live off cancer than die from it.
- Dr. Deepak Chopra

I have not included cancer in the alphabetical listing of diseases and conditions. I do have strong opinions and ideas about the prevention and treatment of cancer, most of which are presented in the ensuing pages, but my hands-on experience has been limited. I do not feel qualified to offer suggestions for treatment. Prevention is another matter. I believe prevention is the only way we can win the ill-named 'war on cancer.' And the way to prevent cancer is to follow the guidelines presented in this book for leading a healthy life-style.

I should hasten to add that there are some cancers that probably cannot be prevented by the measures currently available to us. For while I believe that the majority of cancers fall into our '80%' category (avoidable by consistently making the right lifestyle choices), there are clearly some that are not related to life-style. Think for example of acute leukemia in young children who have not lived long enough for life-style choices to be a factor. There are other rare types of childhood tumors that clearly are not related to factors we currently understand.

In addition, there are certain causative factors that are not related to life-style choices, per se. I am thinking particularly of exposure to toxic substances that we did not know at the time were carcinogenic. When I was a child, we did not know that radiation and asbestos, for example, were carcinogenic agents. I recall happily observing the bones of my feet through the fluoroscope machine in our local shoe store. I am told also that as an infant my thymus gland was irradiated in order to treat my 'breath-holding' spells. Do I consider my survival into old age 'lucky' or is it attributable to the very healthy life-style I've led for the past forty years?

Here is another sad, and to my mind tragic, example: a patient/friend of mine developed an especially horrible and virulent form of cancer. This person lived a very healthy life-style and I knew her well enough to say that she was happy and not under any more stress than the rest of us. A few months after disfiguring surgery and very debilitating chemotherapy and radiation, she died. Her last few weeks were comfortable thanks to the efforts of the staff at an in-patient Hospice unit.

In attempting to find help for her, I asked a colleague of mine if he knew anything about the underlying cause of such a rare malignancy. He asked if it was possible that she had been exposed to heavy metals in her work. I assured him that she had not, but when I asked her about that at a later meeting, she confirmed that she had been quite heavily exposed during the course of her work some ten years previously. Although it was far too late to do anything about it, at least my friend felt some relief knowing that the cancer was not her 'fault.'

Lifestyle is clearly a significant factor for most cancers, especially those which are the current major killers (lung, colon and breast). Most doctors, when patients ask them 'why me' after a diagnosis of cancer, respond with 'it's just the luck of the draw.' I have no patience with practitioners who take that approach. I do understand that some of them are motivated by a desire to avoid blaming the victim, but even then that response is not helpful. In fact, it is often harmful because it leaves the patient with no hope. He or she has no options other than to dutifully follow the so-called 'standard of care': surgery, chemotherapy and radiation. Even if the patient is interested in adopting a healthier life-style after the diagnosis of cancer, there is little opportunity amidst the whirl of treatments, procedures, testing, and more treatments.

It is a radical notion, but I believe that once you have been diagnosed with one of these all-too-common types of cancer, your life-style choices have a lot more to do with your survival and your quality of life than the medical treatments you receive. *But there is a strong caveat here: one man's meat is another man's poison. The choices you make after a diagnosis of cancer have to fit hand-in-glove with what you believe in, or perhaps I should say what you have faith in, in order to enhance your healing.*

For example, if you think that eating organic food and eliminating sugar from your diet is a lot of hogwash, but you do it because your sweet and loving daughter implores you, this choice probably will not help you. If eating brown rice and veggies leaves you feeling deprived and pissed-off, you are better off chowing down on a Big Mac and fries if that is a major source of pleasure for you.

How can I make such a statement when I 'know' that organic foods and a diet low in sugar and trans fats can help prevent cancer? Well, you already have cancer and I don't know you. Sadly, there is no 'proof' yet that these dietary changes increase survival rates. And I don't know what makes you happy. I don't know what you believe in. But hopefully you know these things about yourself and can make the choices that feel right to you.

Why am I talking about happiness and faith? Because the progress of your cancer (as well as prevention of cancer) is dependent mostly on how your immune system is functioning. We are all exposed to carcinogens in our environment – in the food we eat, the water we drink, the air we breathe. Theoretically these substances could cause cancer in any of us, so why do some get cancer and others do not. I do not believe it is the luck of the draw. Rather, it is the optimal functioning of our immune system that defends us against cancer and can assist us in healing from that dread disease.

It is important to look at the factors that enhance our immune functioning and at those that interfere with it. First, let us discuss stress.

Everyone talks about 'stress' as having a negative effect on our immune system, and this is true. We are well adapted to respond to acute stress, but it is commonly thought that modern life puts us into a state of chronic stress, which is deleterious to health. But the more accurate statement is that the things we *experience* as stressful are what are potentially harmful to us. This is a very important distinction. For example, a friend of mine thrives in a chaotic household, where teenagers are coming and going at all hours of the day and night and there is constant disruption and mess in the kitchen and bathrooms. I get tense just being there, and if I had to live in his house, I would be a nervous wreck. It is a 'stressful' environment but he experiences it as pleasant; he feels relaxed and happy at home.

Another example: the death of a spouse is listed as one of the highest possible life stressors. It is not uncommon for the surviving spouse to develop cancer six months to a year after the death of the beloved. On the other hand, I have known women, and men, who have felt a sense of freedom and relief after the death of their spouses and whose health has actually improved.

So, while stress has significant effects on our immune functioning, one must look beneath the surface to determine the importance of a specific event, and this each of us can do for ourselves.

What are other significant factors affecting the functioning of our immune system? The Three Pillars of Health outlined in Chapters 3, 4 and 5 of this book all serve to enhance our immune system. Good nutrition, a sensible exercise program and some form of meditation have all been studied and found to have beneficial effects. In terms of prevention, following this advice will certainly help reduce your chances of developing cancer. If you already have cancer, there is no *proof* that following such a program will improve your long-term survival, but experience and research demonstrate that quality of life is much improved.

Research shows that chronic fear has a profoundly negative effect on the immune system. We have all heard of the flight or fight response that happens during times of an emergency, or more accurately, an *acute* threat to our well being (e.g. an intruder in our home, a tiger in the woods, an out of control vehicle). At those times we either flee the scene or turn and confront the danger with strength we never knew we had. This bodily response produces an increase in the immune response, which aids in our efforts.

On the other hand, when our well-being is *chronically* threatened, as is the case following a diagnosis of cancer, we become fearful and often feel helpless. We experience hopelessness and despair. This is a deadly combination when it comes to immune functioning. And then often we are told that we must endure surgery, chemotherapy and/or radiation, all of which are an assault on our bodies and which seriously interfere with immune functioning.

Many people who work with cancer patients believe that a positive attitude is one of the keys to improved survival. I have no quarrel with this observation, but my in-depth work with patients has taught me that the positive attitude has to be genuine. A bunch of hollow words and phrases will not be helpful to you. If you really have faith in what you are saying, it will be more likely to enhance your health through a beneficial effect on your immune system. Only you can know if you 'really have faith' in something. If you do, you will experience it as an energizing, warm feeling in your body. Others have described it as a 'flow,' or being 'in the zone.' Some scientists go so far as saying that when you are in this state, your molecules are 'happy,' and this of course will be immensely healing.

Are there other ways to make your molecules 'happy?' Certainly, but each person has to find what is right for them. For some, it may be a creative outlet – a special talent you have that you have never taken time to pursue – music, dance, art, writing come to mind but it could be anything that expresses your true self. Or it may be that you want to express a side of yourself that you have kept under wraps; perhaps an aspect of your sexuality, or serving others without concern for remuneration, or living close to nature. There is no end to the possibilities.

Sometimes it is necessary to talk with a counselor or therapist in order to find what is authentic within you and to garner support for what you really want to pursue. Often the people we are closest to, our spouses, siblings, parents and good friends are not supportive of real change in us, especially at a time when we have been diagnosed with a potentially fatal illness. They do not want to lose us. They want us to recover, to heal, and to be happy. And for most of them that means following doctors' orders and living life the way we always have. It will be hard for you to go against that, but it may be necessary in order to save your own life.

How can you do this? How can you find support for taking a path different from the one the doctors and your family want you to follow? It is difficult but I have seen it work. If you elect to make treatment or healing choices that are not truly supported by family and close friends, it will be necessary to develop a network of people who are supportive. Here are some suggestions based on the experience of patients I have known. Find a supportive medical practitioner, such as a family physician who is willing to go out on a limb for you. An 'alternative' practitioner can also be helpful, a trained professional who happens to believe in the body's ability to self-heal. A new friend who has followed a similar path, even if you and this person can only connect by email and phone, can be a very powerful source of support. In short, surround yourself with people who fully accept the healing choices you have made.

I have avoided a discussion of specific unconventional or alternative treatments when it comes to cancer, because that is not the purpose of this book. But I will emphasize that whatever approach fits with your belief system – in other words, that which you have faith in – is likely to be of benefit to your well-being and to your survival.

There is one final observation that I feel I must include in this brief discussion of cancer. It is not something that I have read about in books and articles dealing with cancer and no other doctors have ever mentioned it to me. I have known several men and women who apparently have chosen cancer as a way to escape a life they can no longer tolerate. I use the word apparently, but in two instances, the patients have told me that this was the case. In both instances the individual could not face living any longer with his/her spouse, but could not or would not muster up the courage to leave the marriage. And ironically, in both of these situations, the spouse became a devoted caretaker of the patient in his/her final months of life. In the other instances, the truth about the relationship was unspoken but quite obvious to anyone knowing the intimate details of the person's marriage.

Why do I include this dreadfully disheartening observation? Could it possibly be of help to anyone? My hope is that if this scenario fits for you, that you will find a way to speak the truth to your wife or husband. It is a hunch, but I do not think you will have to leave the marriage. If you and your spouse are willing to focus on the true nature of your relationship and to get some professional help with it, I believe that process could be life-saving. In that process, some very strong feelings will arise within you, and if you give free rein to those emotions, they can assist you in your recovery.

It is worth repeating again: when energy and feeling flow freely through the body, immune functioning is optimized, laying the groundwork for healing.

Part III – Resources for Self Cure: Exercises, Meditations and Diet

The resources in Part III are intended for use by those who have read Part I and the relevant chapters in Part II. These exercises and techniques will aid you in the pursuit of health and disease prevention. Throughout this book we have emphasized the importance of self-awareness. By getting to really know yourself physically, mentally, emotionally and spiritually, you will then be in a position to know which of the methods described in this book will be helpful to you personally. Some of the exercises are easy, others more difficult to master. Be patient with yourself.

If you are new to these types of exercises, start very slowly, a few minutes per day. Whether it is a breathing exercise, a relaxation technique, or a dietary change, take enough time to find out if it fits with your way of being in the world, with your age, your health problems and your goals for yourself. None of these exercises by themselves should be considered a to be a cure for a specific condition. They must be done in concert with the three pillars of good health and with the advice given in the section pertaining to your problem or condition, including the warnings of when it is paramount to seek medical attention.

It is not my intention to make the exercises and techniques sound onerous. To the contrary, if they fit for you, they will be a pleasure to perform – once you learn them - and a source of joy in your busy day.

45 BREATH AND VOICE EXERCISES

With visible breath I am walking. A voice I am sending as I walk. In a sacred manner I am walking.
- Black Elk

1)   Calming Breath for Mind and Body

- Sit in a straight-backed chair with both feet flat on the floor and your eyes closed.

- Bring your awareness to the sounds in the environment for a moment or two.

- Now bring your awareness to your body for a moment or two.

- Sigh deeply with mouth open or closed, releasing the air in your lungs. Let the new breath come in naturally. Repeat 3 times.

- Inhale lifting your shoulders up to your ears. Hold for a second or two and then release the breath letting the shoulders sink at the same time.

- Inhale again lifting your shoulders up; this time squeeze the shoulders into the base of the skull and hold both your shoulders and your breath for several seconds. Release the breath and the shoulders very slowly, encouraging the shoulders to sink way down as if the shoulder blades are sliding down your back. At the same time feel your head floating upward.

- Next, with each breath, extend the length of the exhale by a second or two. Let your inhalations be slow and comfortably deep. Notice the pause at the end of each exhale before the inhale starts again and become aware of the pause at the end of each inhale just before the exhale begins. Over time, try to make your exhalations considerably longer than your inhalations.

Practice for 5 minutes at first, several times a day. After a few days, you will be able to perform this technique with ease and pleasure. You will also find that you can adapt it to stressful situations, even in public.

2)   Sleep promoting Breath

- Lying in bed, breathe out fully, then breathe in very slowly until your lungs feel comfortably full.

- Then hold the breath in without straining for as long as you are able to stay relaxed – especially the throat muscles and glottis (try to work up to 30 seconds).

- Release the breath slowly through your mouth, making a 'shhushhing' sound.

- Rest for about ten seconds,

- Repeat the process three to five more times.

You may discover that you have fallen asleep after a couple of repetitions.

3) Energizing Breath (aka Bellows Breath) for Mind and Body

Standing in the Basic Stance position (Chapter 46, number 1), breathe out forcefully and rapidly through the nose, letting the in-breath flow naturally (without force) into your lungs. You will feel your diaphragm and belly "pump" with each forced out breath. Do 25-30 of these breaths in rapid succession.

The first few times you try this you may become dizzy due to rapid changes in your blood chemistry. Slow down until you become used to it. If you wish, you can energize even more by using your arms like a bird's wings – place your fists next to your shoulders, forming a 'wing' and flap like a bird (or bellows) with each out breath.

4) General Health promoting Breath (aka Great Circle Breath)

Do this exercise outside in the fresh air, early in the morning, facing the rising sun.

- Stand in the Basic Stance position (Chapter 46, number 1) with your arms relaxed and hands cupped in front of you at the level of your pelvis.

- From their midline position, slowly raise your hands up and out to the side in an arc, as if making a big circle around your upper body.

- As you raise the hands, inhale slowly through the nose or mouth until your hands meet at the top and your lungs are full of fresh air.

- Hold the posture and the breath for 5 – 10 seconds. Then, place one hand on top of the other (both palms facing downward) and slowly 'press' the hands downward in front of your body as you exhale. Imagine you are pumping the air out of your lungs.

- When your hands reach their original position at your pelvis, remain standing and resting for 5 – 10 seconds. Then repeat the whole process again and do this 6 – 12 times.

- End the exercise by folding into the Hanging Over posture (Exercise 1, Chapter 46) and rest there for about 15 seconds.

5) Basic Voice Exercise (the Big AHHHHH)

Lie on a carpeted floor or a firm mat and place a rolled-up bath towel under your shoulder blades so that your back is slightly arched and your head tilted back. Aim for an 'open' feeling in your chest. Bend your knees so that your feet rest flat against the carpet.

- Now, open your mouth wide, keeping the lower jaw relaxed. Take a moderately deep breath into your belly, hold it for two seconds, then release it with a loud, clear, sustained sound. Do not force the sound. Imagine you have opened your mouth wide for the doctor to examine your throat. Say AHHHHHH, but make it loud and clear and long. Let the sound pour out of you, as the water flows from the faucet in your bathtub. Strive for freedom in the sound of your voice. Let it flow to the very end of your breath, until there is no air left in your lungs.

- Rest for about five seconds and then repeat the process, doing at least ten repetitions.

With daily practice, you will be able to sustain the AHHHH sound for 30-50 seconds, thus opening your voice and increasing your lung capacity at the same time.

6) Assertive Voice Exercise

This is an excellent exercise for those of you who have problems asserting yourselves in the world. It will help to mobilize your healthy aggression. It is necessary to master the Basic Voice Exercise (above) before attempting this one. Stand in the Basic Stance position (Chapter 46, number 1). Place your fists on your hips, pull your pelvis and elbows back slightly so that your chest puffs out a bit.

- Focus your eyes on a spot on the wall across from you and direct your voice and your energy (through your eyes) toward that spot.
- Use the technique in exercise 5, releasing the voice clear and loud.
- Imagine your voice and your energy hitting that spot like a laser beam, sending it up in smoke.
- Be sure to keep yourself grounded to the floor as you release the sound – stand tall and firm. Do not waiver or collapse in mind or body. Repeat the process ten times.

7) Singing

If you love to sing and do so frequently, in a loud, clear voice, you probably don't need any other voice exercise. To maximize the health benefits of your singing, follow these guidelines.

- Sing with an 'open throat.' This does not mean forcing the voice; rather, it means letting it flow (see above under basic voice exercise) in a clear, unconstricted, uninhibited manner.
- Try to match the song, both the tune and the lyrics, to whatever you are feeling at the time. You can even make up words to familiar melodies to express your sadness, or longing or anger and hopefully, at times, your joy.
- Sing for at least ten minutes every day.

46 FLEXIBILITY EXERCISES

*Yoga teaches us to cure what need not be
endured and endure what cannot be cured.*
- B.K.S. Iyengar

The two exercises described below, when mastered,
will give you improved flexibility throughout your body
and enhance the flow of feeling and energy through
your body. Even if you are taking yoga classes, these
two exercises will enhance your performance.

1) Grounding Exercise (Basic Stance and Bend)

*This exercise is a prerequisite to all the other flexibility and
expressive exercises that follow. It will give you a strong sense of
Self and a feeling of deep connection with the ground beneath you.
It will help to keep you calm, centered and focused.*

Do this exercise in bare feet, standing on a wooden
floor, a carpet or outside on the lawn. Stand with your
feet parallel to each other and about ten inches apart.

- Bend your knees slightly (just so they are not locked) and shift your weight gently toward the balls of your feet. Your heels should remain firmly on the ground.

- Relax your feet and legs so that you can feel more contact with the earth/floor beneath you. Feel the support it is giving you.

- Let your pelvis 'hang' in the midline - that is, neither thrust forward nor pulled back. Think of a pendulum which has come to rest at the bottom of its swing.

- Throughout the exercise, keep your attention on your connection with the earth. Now, straighten your spine and stand tall. Keep your head level and relax your jaw so that your mouth hangs open a bit. Let your hands hang loosely at your sides. If possible, also let your belly hang by releasing the abdominal muscles.

- Stand this way for three to five minutes, breathing freely and openly. Keep your eyes relaxed and soft, gazing off into the distance.

- Remember to keep your attention on the connection between your feet and the ground. As you stand, you may notice some shaking in the muscles of your legs. This is normal and desirable and should be encouraged. It is simply a release of tension.

After three to five minutes, go into the "Bend" or "Hanging Over" step as follows:

- Keeping your weight on the balls of your feet, slowly let yourself hang forward from the hips (not the waist). Remember to keep the knees slightly bent.

- Let your arms hang loosely in front of you. If your hands actually reach the floor, place your fingertips lightly on the ground. It is very important to drop your head while in this position, so that the top of your head is parallel to the ground.

- Relax into this position and maintain it for 30 to 60 seconds. As you stay in the bend, you may notice that the shaking in your legs intensifies. If so, this is a good sign.

To end the exercise, let yourself all the way down to the floor and rest for awhile on your belly or back.

2) Basic Energizing Exercise

To bring a feeling of vibrancy and energy into the body, do the standing and bending over exercise as described above. Then, instead of dropping to the floor and resting, bring yourself back into the standing position in this manner:

- Keep the weight forward on the balls of your feet and slowly straighten your spine until you are standing again. As you come up out of the hanging over position, it is important to let your head hang until you are fully erect. Also, to avoid feeling lightheaded, take several noisy, rapid breaths on your way up.

- Now that you are back in the standing position, place your palms in the small of your back and arch slightly backwards, so that the front of your body is stretched somewhat. As you do this, keep your feet firmly rooted to the floor. Also, keep your eyes open and focused on a distant point.

- Hold this posture for about 30 to 60 seconds while making the AHHHHH sound described above. Then, ease back into the basic stance and drop slowly over into the bend.

- Do three to five repetitions of this technique. You will probably notice that the shaking in your legs becomes more intense, indicating that you are releasing more tension.

- Finally, just stand in the basic stance position, breathing freely and easily through your mouth. Release any sound that feels right to you.

With practice, you will feel energy surging through your body. Do not be surprised if emotions well up while you are doing the exercise – simply let them flow without judgment while you stay grounded in the basic stance – they will subside naturally.

If you are unable to experience the vibrating sensation created during this exercise, an acceptable alternative is to bounce gently on a mini-trampoline (e.g. a Rebounder) for ten minutes. Your feet do not have to leave the surface. Let the muscles of your body relax as much as possible while you are bouncing - loosen your jaw, shoulders and belly. Breathe freely through your mouth, hum or otherwise vocalize while you bounce.

47 EXPRESSIVE EXERCISES

Parents, teach your children to express themselves. Teach them to be in touch with their emotions, to speak honestly to people, and to maintain integrity and stick by their principles in all they do. This is perhaps the highest morality you can instill. But don't expect them to succeed in business.
- Jeffrey Bryant

1) Laughing

Research has shown that laughing is a very health-enhancing activity. What is most interesting is that the benefits accrue whether or not the laugh is 'genuine.' In other words, self-induced or exercise laughing is just as healthful as the real thing. This should be good news to those of you who are depressed and/or in chronic pain and find it hard to be amused by comedy. On a personal note, I grew up as a very serious young man. I rarely laughed. I began in my forties practicing an exercise routine that included laughing each day. Within a few months, I found that I was laughing out loud in social situations and at genuinely funny comedies. Moreover, my sense of humor in all situations improved markedly. Yes, I am still a serious person, but not at all grim.

Laugh out loud for ten minutes each day. No matter how you feel, start with making the ha-ha-ha sound, even if you have to fake and force it. You all know what raucous laughter sounds like, so aim for that. Do it sitting, standing, or lying down, whatever makes it easier for you to get the sound out. Please do not try to do other tasks while laughing, except perhaps for showering or driving the car, which are automatic tasks and will not take your mind off the laughter. Keep this up on a daily basis for at least two weeks before you decide that it is not doing you any good. Remember that even if it does not improve your mood, the exercise is very helpful to your immune system and thereby is useful in health promotion and disease prevention.

2) Crying

Crying as an exercise is rarely mentioned in any of the articles and books I have read on healing. Yet in my work with patients I have found it to be a very valuable tool especially for people who say they hardly ever cry. *If you are a person who cries easily, especially when someone hurts you, this exercise is not for you. I encourage you to move on to the anger releasing exercises below.*

When I say crying, I do not mean leaking tears, which we shall refer to as weeping. By crying I mean all out sobbing (boo-hoo) with sound and energy. When you sob, the diaphragm moves fully and energy flows freely up and down the body. If you doubt this, watch a small child cry openly. Also note that after a "good cry," the body relaxes and there is a tendency to feel sleepy.

Try this crying exercise when you are feeling hurt and sad and perhaps are weeping, but can't seem to really cry/sob.

- Lie flat on the floor or on a firm bed and place a small pillow under your neck.
- Bend your knees so your feet rest flat against the floor or bed (this loosens the abdominal muscles).
- Open your mouth wide and make an ah-ah-ah-ah sound, trying to imitate the sound of sobbing. Keep it up for a couple of minutes until actual sobbing takes over.

  If it helps, pound your fists into the floor as you sob.

Sometimes it helps to say a word, loud, over and over, like 'please' or 'why.' If you are lucky enough to get to spontaneous sobbing, let it run its course until it subsides naturally. Then rest a few minutes before getting up.

3) Releasing Anger:

There are many safe ways to release the anger that has built up inside you. This is important so that it does not poison you or others in your environs. Remember that I have said that freely expressed adult anger is useful and transient. It is the chronically held anger and resentment and hostility which results in seething, which is bad for your health. So next time you realize that you are seething, try any of the anger releasing exercises listed below. In every one of them, the release of sound via the voice is just as important as the physical movements.

a) Pounding: This exercise is the one most preferred by my patients. When done correctly and regularly, it will result in the letting go of chronically held anger within a few weeks. Minimal equipment is needed: an old tennis racket or child's plastic baseball bat and several old firm cushions. Pile the cushions on top of a high bed or low table until the top one is level with your waist. Stand in front of the table at a distance that allows you to freely smack the cushions with the bat. Ground yourself by standing in the basic stance (Chapter 46, number 1). Raise the bat straight above your head so the tip of it is pointing towards the ceiling. Keeping your shoulders loose, smack the cushions with the bat. As you do this, take care not to bend from the waist. If necessary, bend your knees with each blow to enhance the force. Each time the bat hits the cushions, make a loud sound with your voice. Any expressive sound will do. Examples include the Karate 'hah' or NO or any single syllable curse word that feels satisfying to you. Be sure to take in a breath before each hit. Start out by hitting the cushions 25 times, and then add a few hits each day until you work up to 100.

b) Kicking: This exercise is especially useful for those of you who have an urge to kick things. It will help to release the anger stored in the muscles of your legs. Lie on a very firm bed or thick mat with a thin pillow beneath your head. Begin by bending your right knee fully and then raising the foot toward the ceiling; try to do this in a smooth, fluid motion. Next bring the leg straight down forcefully so that your heel and the entire length of the back of the leg strike the mat at the same time. As soon as your right leg hits the mat, begin raising the left leg in preparation for the kick. Do this slowly at first, alternating legs. Release the voice each time your leg hits the mat (see above under Pounding). As you get used to the process, speed it up until it feels like a satisfying release. Continue kicking until you are fatigued, then rest flat on the bed for a few minutes. Most people can work up to 100 kicks over the course of a few days.

c) Destruction: This is a very satisfying exercise, especially when your anger has been triggered by another person and there is nothing you can safely do about it. It involves the use of all muscles of your body that are mobilized for a good fight.

Find a medium size sturdy cardboard box and place it open side down on the table you use for the pounding exercise (see above). Use the bat to smash the box as much as you can. Then throw the box on the floor and flatten it some more by stomping on it with your feet. Then pick it up and tear it to shreds with your hands. When the pieces get too small to tear, use your teeth to further destroy them. As much as possible, release the voice with curses, howls, and growls. When you are finished with your destruction, sit quietly and look at the pile of rubble before you clean it up. Notice how you feel.

d)   Crazy Talk: A better word for this exercise is gibberish. It is extremely effective for those times when you can't get the negative thinking to stop. When done correctly, the exercise will clear your mind and lift your mood. It takes practice to get it 'right.' Stand in front of the mirror and look intently at your image. Imagine that he or she is someone you can trust with all your feelings. Begin by talking nonsense slowly, continuing to look at the person in the mirror. By nonsense or gibberish I mean that what you are saying makes no sense whatsoever. Do not use any real words at all. If you have trouble getting started, say 'abadabadababada' over and over until some other nonsense words start flowing out of your mouth spontaneously. The non-words should come from your body, not your brain. Babble like an infant, rave like a lunatic. Use hand and facial gestures to facilitate the expression of emotion. Keep going for at least five minutes.

48 BRAIN EXERCISE

It shouldn't be surprising that the brain
benefits from exercise like the rest of the body,
maybe even more.
- Ian Robertson

This very specific exercise will help boost your brain power. Sit in a straight backed chair with your hands on your lap, palms upward. On each hand at the same time, touch the tips of your thumb and your forefinger together briefly, then move on to the thumb and middle finger, thumb and ring finger and thumb and pinky. Then return to thumb and forefinger, etc. This should be a steady, rhythmic percussion, as slow or as fast as you need to keep it going without losing track or missing fingers. When you get the hang of it, add the voice component (an ancient chant derived from Sanskrit) as follows: Starting with the forefinger touch, say SA; with middle, TA; with ring, say NA; with pinky, say MA. SA-TA-NA-MA, SA-TA-NA-MA, etc. over and over with the rhythm of your finger touch. Keep this up for seven minutes. When you are finished, close your eyes and sit quietly for a moment.

49 SEXUAL EXERCISES

People that are exercising and eating a good diet do have sex more frequently and do have less problems with sexual dysfunction and those types of problems.
- Dr. Charles Rice

It is worth repeating here that these exercises work best in conjunction with your efforts to correct the underlying causes of your lack of sexual desire or impotence. Please see the section on sexual exercise in Chapter 4 of this book, and also Chapter 27 - Impotence. The sexual exercises detailed below are designed to free up chronic tension in the pelvis and/or to stimulate the flow of energy in the sexual organs. Each of these exercises should be done on a daily basis for at least a month in order to enhance sexual energy.

1) Sesame Oil Self-Massage

This is an exercise from the Ayurvedic tradition. Use refined sesame oil, which is odorless and non-greasy. Before your morning shower or bath, treat yourself to a slow, sensuous total body massage in a very warm bathroom.

2) Lower abdominal rubbing

Lying flat on your back use the palm of your hand to rub your lower belly in a circular motion. Start with the right hand – exert enough pressure as you rub to create a sensation of warmth in the area below your navel down to the pubic bone. Take your time, keep your attention on your hand and your belly, rub slowly and firmly. Make 50- 100 circles. Then switch hands and use your left hand to make circles in the opposite direction.

3) Pelvic Bounce

Lie on the floor or a firm mat with a small pillow under your head. Place a rolled up towel under the small of your back (the roll should be no more than three inches thick). Bend your knees so your feet are flat against the mat. Using your leg muscles, push into the mat with your feet so your pelvis is lifted slightly (one to two inches) off the mat. Then let it drop to the mat. Try to avoid using your abdominal or pelvic muscles to lift the pelvis; let the movement come from your feet. Repeat the lifting and dropping movement rapidly and as freely and easily as you can. Keep breathing and/or making a sound of pleasure as you bounce the pelvis against the mat. Do at least 100 bounces, 200 if possible.

4) Squeeze and release

In the same position as above, separate your feet and knees about 15 inches. Place a rubber ball (soccer ball size is perfect) between your knees and squeeze the ball as tightly as you can for at least ten seconds. Then suddenly release the tension, letting the ball drop. Feel the letting go in the pelvis. Repeat this process of squeeze and release at least ten times.

5) Anal lock

Lie on your back in bed or on the floor. Stretch your legs out fully. Raise your big toes towards your head without moving your feet or legs. At the same time, squeeze your anus shut as tightly as possible. Hold the squeeze for five to ten seconds. Continue to breathe freely as you do this. Repeat the exercise ten times.

6) Hopping

This exercise is similar to using a trampoline. In fact, if you own a mini trampoline or 'Rebounder' and feel safe on it, use that. Standing naked in a warm room, raise your arms straight above your head, palms pointing toward each other. Now, bend your knees slightly and execute a very small jump; you do not even need to clear the floor as long as the feeling is one of jumping or hopping, a movement which 'jiggles' your whole body. With each jump, pump your fists; that is, squeeze your hands shut and open them fully. Make sure that this exercise is not causing pain in your knees or back (if so, discontinue its use). Hop 50 to 100 times.

50 MEDITATION, VISUALIZATION AND IMAGERY TECHNIQUES

Meditation increases your vitality and strengthens your intelligence; your beauty is enhanced; your mental clarity and health improve.
— Mata Amritanandamayi ("Amma")

The goal of the meditative and other techniques described here is to promote health and prevent disease. They are mind/body techniques and have no particular religious or spiritual bases.

This section describes several varieties of meditative exercises and techniques which can be very helpful to you for your overall health and well-being, for obtaining symptom relief, and for healing from specific diseases and conditions. *However, before attempting any of these, please read Chapter 5 - Going to the Source in Part I of this book and practice the basic technique described there.*

1) Mantra Meditation

The technique described in Part I is one form of mantra meditation. There are many others. For example, you can substitute another word or short phrase for the word "one." I encourage people with a religious background to use a snippet of prayer such as "Thy will be done," or parts of the Rosary. For others, a line from a soothing nursery rhyme or lullaby works well ("The world is so full of a number of things......"). Yoga students may prefer a Sanskrit word that has a soothing tone when repeated over and over. The important thing to keep in mind is that it is not the meaning of the word or phrase that is important. Rather, it is the effect that the repetition has on your mind and body.

2) Mindfulness

There are many excellent books written on the subject of Mindfulness Meditation. However, for our purposes, I will describe a simple mindfulness or 'awareness' technique that will be useful for mental and physical health and well-being.

Begin with a few minutes of the basic technique described in Chapter 5, then, while maintaining the correct posture, give your mind free rein to go wherever it goes while you continue to sit and observe the process. This is very different from thinking, which is a purposeful creation of thoughts, usually with a goal of solving something (such as what am I going to make for dinner or why do I hate my boss). With mindfulness, you observe what is going on in your mind (and body) as if you were watching a movie – in other words, you are somewhat detached from what is happening. Keep this up for approximately 20 minutes, then end by returning to the breath.

By observing your thoughts, emotions and bodily responses in this manner, you will gradually learn more about yourself, your authentic self, than you ever dreamed was possible. Self-awareness is the best tool you can possess in order to self-heal. When you truly become adept at this (it may take years), you can throw away this book.

3) Chanting

While not strictly a meditation technique, chanting can be very calming to the mind and body if done correctly. You must first learn the chant from a book or CD. Choose one in which the actual sounds are soothing to your ear; do not look for something 'meaningful.' For example, sitting and chanting the Rosary out loud for ten or twenty minutes, without giving any thought to the meaning of the words, enables many people to get through a stressful day. For others, a Sanskrit chant works best. Note that this process is not the same as singing (see Voice exercises).

4) Walking Meditation

You can kill two birds with one stone' by using this technique correctly. You will be exercising your body in a healthful way and doing a meditation technique at the same time. It is especially useful for those of you who are pressed for time each day. There are some prerequisites. First, you must have the experience of the basic meditation technique described in Chapter 5. Second, you must walk in a safe place; that is, not on a busy street. Good locations are the outdoor tracks at your local high school (when it is not being used for other purposes), quiet country roads, or suburban streets in the early morning. I do not recommend mall-walking because of the poor quality of the indoor recycled air. Third, you must walk alone.

Walk at a steady, moderate pace. Fix your eyes on a point in the distance. Become acutely aware of the sensation of your feet contacting the ground with each step. Establish a rhythm that you can feel coursing through your body. Match your breathing to that rhythm; however that works best for you. For example, it might be four steps with each in-breath and four steps with each out-breath. Or, two steps with each in-breath and four steps with each out-breath. Of course, it has to be an even number because we have two feet.

After you learn to do this and it becomes (probably after a few days) a routine, add the third component, as follows. Add a 'sub-vocal' recitation of even numbered syllables. This is not as complex as it sounds. Cadets learn to march to the sound of 'hup-two-three-four, hup-two-three-four.' If you were to sub-vocalize this, it would be breathing in to the mental sound of hup-two, and breathing out to the sound of three-four. One recitation that I made up years ago was "I am good and I am strong I can walk here all day long."

Once you have mastered this technique, it becomes easy and pleasant to do and the time passes very quickly. Before you know it, you have walked for twenty minutes or a half hour, covered perhaps a mile and a half, and returned home in a good frame of mind and with an energized body. This is the opposite of what happens to people when they go out for a walk and think about their problems.

51 USING IMAGERY AND VISUALIZATION TO HEAL SPECIFIC PROBLEMS AND CONDITIONS

Diseases of the soul are more dangerous and more numerous than those of the body.
- Cicero

We have seen how unexpressed emotions can get 'stuck' in the body, causing areas of chronic tension and blocks to the free flow of energy. When this state persists, we often develop somatic symptoms and even diseases. Many of the voice and body exercises described above are designed to open those blocks and prevent the development of disease states.

We can also use the power of the conscious mind to assist in overcoming our mental and physical health problems. I am not talking here about changing our belief system through the power of positive thinking, although that approach has been helpful to many and I encourage you to explore it elsewhere if you wish. The techniques described below have nothing to do with 'thinking.' Rather, they are exercises in 'seeing' things differently. And it has been wisely said that if one can see things differently, one will be able to do things a new way.

The only skill required to practice these techniques is the innate ability that most of us have to visualize things in our mind's eye. Some people are much more adept than others at visualization; I myself am at the lower end of the continuum but have nevertheless benefited greatly from the practice.

Close your eyes and visualize a lemon. If you can see it clearly – its shape, color, size – and can hold that image for as long as you desire, you are an excellent candidate for these techniques.

1) Healing Psychological Traumas

Sit in the meditative posture, with your eyes closed. Visualize the traumatic event (make it as specific as possible) and notice your emotional and bodily response to seeing it happen. Let us say that it is your step-father in your bedroom, looking at you with hatred in his eyes and then beating you with a leather belt. Now, let go of that image and breathe out fully three times. Now see yourself in the same room at the same age with your step-father, but he is looking at you with kindness in his eyes and asking you about your day, then perhaps tucking you in, saying goodnight, and turning out the light. In other words, 'see' it happen the way you wish it could have been, the way that would have been nourishing to you. See this new scene unfolding for 30-60 seconds and notice the effect on you body. Then breathe out again and get up from the chair. See this new, healing scene in your mind's eye 5 to 10 times over the course of the day for several weeks.

2) Dispelling Rage - an End to 'Seething'

This technique can be done in conjunction with the anger-releasing physical exercise techniques (see above) or by itself. It will be especially useful to those of you with ailments that preclude the use of the more vigorous physical exercises.

Sit in the meditative posture with your eyes closed. Feel the rage in your body and see the images that accompany the emotion. Let us say that you are enraged at your boss for treating you unfairly and perhaps with disdain or contempt. See him standing in front of you in the office. Notice all the details of his appearance and of the room you are in. Then, see yourself becoming as big and strong as the Hulk or The Terminator or your favorite fantastically powerful character and see yourself using your strength and your aggression to do whatever you wish to the boss in order to feel satisfied. When you are satisfied, notice the effect on your body. Let go of the image and sit quietly for a minute or two.

3) Dumping Your Problems

This works well when you can't stop ruminating or perseverating about your problems. You just can't get those worrisome thoughts out of your head.

Sit in the meditative posture. Imagine using a broom or shovel to make a huge pile of all your problems in a field at the edge of a cliff. Now use a bulldozer to push that pile over the edge of the cliff, where they fall to a bottomless ravine. Climb down off the bulldozer, dust off your hands, and walk away in the sunshine.

4) Decision Making

I have never had much luck trying to decide on this versus that based on logic or reason. Making lists of the pros and cons and weighting them with stars or numbers has never been really helpful to me. I devised this imagery technique which has been immensely useful to me and to many of my patients.

Sit in a meditative posture and bring your attention to the decision at hand. Let's keep it simple and say you are in a store trying to decide between two equally beautiful new dresses. Close your eyes and see yourself going out to dinner at your favorite restaurant in dress A. Be sure to see the dining room clearly and the other people you are with. Notice your bodily reaction as you see this. Next, breathe out and let go of that image. Breathe out again and now see yourself in dress B in the same location. Again, notice your bodily reaction. Chances are your body will tell you which one to choose.

You can use this process to make more serious, even major decisions, such as whether to leave your marriage. But you must see yourself clearly in the both situations, without words or thoughts.

The more specific you can be, the better it will work. See yourself in a certain room at a specific time of day. See what you are doing. Let the scene unfold and notice how you feel, physically and emotionally. Then imagine yourself in the alternative situation, again very specifically, and notice your reactions. Let your decisions come from your body.

52 ANTI-INFLAMMATORY DIET

Let food be thy medicine and medicine be thy food.
- Hippocrates

Whether your health is currently compromised or you just want to experiment to find out if you could feel better on a different diet, the anti-inflammatory diet presented here[6] can be useful. Bear in mind that following the 7 Guidelines for Eating Well in Chapter 3 should reduce inflammation considerably. This more strict diet is available when that's not enough (for example, when facing a cancer diagnosis or during an acute flare-up of rheumatoid arthritis or other autoimmune disorders).

---

[6] My wife and I [Stormon] discovered this diet when she was stricken with breast cancer. Faced with a life-threatening illness, we researched extensively, and found evidence for diet's role in promoting or preventing cancer and a host of other maladies. My wife still follows this diet (most of the time) as a general health measure and she is healthier than she has ever been in her life.

Trying this diet for 21 days (three full weeks) is a good place to start. During this time, don't allow yourself "treats" or other deviations from the diet. Strict adherence is the only way to really know how this will affect you. Trigger foods, even in very small quantities can cause issues for up to two weeks, so for this diet to work, it is important not to cheat, and to stick with it.

You may find that you feel much better after following this diet, but that you miss certain foods after 21 days. If you add foods back (one at a time!) and pay careful attention to the effects, you can build your own list of trigger foods to avoid. Sometimes it is the cumulative effects of foods in the "avoid completely" category, so it is not always possible to nail down single or exact causes. If you are facing a serious illness, it might be better to just stick to the diet.

Let's start with what you can eat:
  a. Pasture-raised, hormone-free beef, chicken, turkey, or lamb.
  b. Organic free-range eggs (include both yolk and white).
  c. Try to eat only wild and not farm raised fish.
  d. After the first week, you may add organic whole milk from pasture-raised cows, sheep, or goats. If you notice any reaction, stop immediately.
  e. All the fresh organic non-starchy non-nightshade vegetables you want. Of course if you are allergic to any vegetable, do not include it.

f.   Up to one fresh, raw, organic apple per day (or the equivalent volume in berries) eaten after a meal.

g.   Organic butter, extra-virgin olive oil, coconut oil and fats that naturally exist on the meats you are eating (leave the skin on the chicken, yolk in the egg, etc.)

h.   Any kind of organic raw nuts or seeds. Soak these overnight in water, throw away the water and use immediately, dehydrate or refrigerate. Don't include if you are allergic.

i.   Stevia.

j.   Fresh or dried organic herbs and spices.

k.   Plenty of spring, well or filtered water between meals.

Sounds pretty tasty, right? OK, now the more difficult news. Here's what you have to completely avoid in order for this to work:

a.   No packaged or fast food, pork, luncheon meats, hot dogs, sausages.

b.   No egg beaters or other egg-like substitutes.

c.   No shark, swordfish, tuna, blue fish, orange roughy or farm-raised fish like tilapia.

d.   No dairy products including milk, cheese, yogurt, cream, cream cheese, cottage cheese, ice cream, etc.

e.   No frozen, dried, canned, packaged or processed vegetables and no starchy vegetables (such as corn, potatoes, yams, winter squash) of any kind. No nightshade vegetables such as eggplant, potatoes, tomatoes or bell peppers. That includes anything made from potatoes.

f. No grains (rice, wheat, oats, etc.) or grain products including flour, breads, pastas, noodles, cereals, crackers. No beans or bean products.

g. No fruit juices of any kind. No sports drinks, flavored water, soda, energy drink or anything but water.

h. No other fats and oils including mayonnaise, salad dressings, canola, soybean, safflower, cottonseed etc.

i. No sweeteners other than Stevia. No sugar, honey, molasses, brown rice syrup, corn syrup, fruit sweeteners, maple syrup, or artificial sweeteners.

j. No nuts or seeds which have been roasted, salted, honey coated, wasabi-coated nuts, etc.

k. No packaged spice combinations.

l. No caffeine or alcohol.

53 SOFTENING THE BELLY AND PELVIC FLOOR

*I am the Belly, I am the mothership, I am the
door to your mother's womb. I am the body
erotic, electric. I create, procreate, recreate. I
am excessive. Wild celebration. In me hides
unbounded aliveness, appetite for the
unknown, mysterious calls of longing and
fulfillment.*
-Margot Anand, The Art of Everyday Ecstasy

It is very common to have tightness in the belly and
in the pelvic floor. In fact, exercise programs are touted
to give us a "tight" belly. They are shooting for core
strength and good abdominal muscle tone which are
important. Here I'm referring to tightness which
restricts movement and the free flow of energy. You
may not even notice this tightness, but I encourage you
to try these exercises and see what you experience.

1) Softening the Belly

Sit comfortably with your hands on your belly. Breathe deeply and feel the warmth of your hands. Gently and lovingly massage your belly, imagining the heat of your hands relaxing tensions and healing whatever needs it. Allow the belly to rise naturally with each inhale and soften with each exhale. Think to yourself, "let go" or "it's alright" and notice any images, thoughts or feelings which come up.

It's possible that you will encounter resistance or strong feelings as you do this exercise. If so, take a break and try it again another time. But do keep practicing until you can easily soften your belly whenever you intend to. Then start noticing times during the day when your belly tightens. Does it happen when something feels threatening or when you feel ashamed of your shape and "suck in" your belly? How about when you are expected to perform? Experiment with softening your belly at these times and notice if you feel more energy and a greater ability to respond to and flow with the situation.

2) Softening the Pelvic Floor

Once you have mastered softening your belly, you are ready to learn to relax the area of the body known as the pelvic floor. These are the muscles and connective tissues that support the genitals and anus. Learning to consciously soften this area can provide a great deal of benefit.

Lie on your back with your neck supported by a pillow or rolled up towel, knees bent and the soles of the feet on the floor. Close your eyes, soften your belly and then bring attention to your pelvic floor. Breathe deeply and notice the connection between your breath and the pelvic floor. You may be able to feel the softening and broadening of the pelvic floor with each inhalation and a gentle drawing up or contraction of the pelvic floor as you exhale.

Now accentuate these natural actions. Gently expand your pelvic floor muscles by pushing out and down, and then follow with a contraction, drawing in and up. Coordinate this with your breathing in whatever way feels comfortable to you. Keep the belly soft. Feel free to place your hands on your pelvic muscles to help you feel what's going on. If you encounter tightness, keep breathing while gently massaging the area until it softens. Check to make sure that you are still breathing deeply, that your belly is still soft and that your mouth and jaw are relaxed. It's also fine to make any sounds that come up or feel right.

You may observe strong emotions or negative thoughts coming up. Just observe these without judgment. It's fine to take a break and start again later. It may also be helpful to try the corresponding expressive exercises from Chapter 47. This technique is complementary to the pelvic exercises found in Chapter 49 as well as to the pelvic release work described in Chapter 29.

ABOUT THE AUTHORS

Mark J. Sicherman, M.D. practiced pediatrics in the Army, in private practice and clinic settings for about 12 years. He went on to study MindBody Medicine and after 5 years of training, supervision and therapy at the New York Society for Bioenergetic Analysis, Dr. Sicherman was certified as a bioenergetic therapist. This was a life-altering experience for him personally and for his practice. For the next 35 years Dr. Sicherman worked with adult patients, practicing with them the kind of medicine he has written about in this book. Dr. Sicherman and his wife live on the beautiful farm which she found for them nearly forty years ago in Upstate New York.

Chuck Stormon is a father of two and a serial entrepreneur with a master's degree in computer engineering. During his wife's diagnosis and treatment for breast cancer Mr. Stormon became her supporter, researcher and health advocate. They discovered and continue to practice the vital health enhancing principals and techniques presented in this book. The Stormons live with their cat in Upstate New York enjoying good friends, farm fresh food and abundant trees, lakes and waterfalls.